In the last decade or so there has been a quiet epidemic in temperate lands of the m

condition. Previously active, health exhausted shadows with br is happening to them? The licity about this condition, flu', post viral fatigue synd drome, Royal Free disease, or myalgic litis – ME. There have been conflicting and confusing headlines; is it 'all in the mind'?, is it a persisting viral infection?, or is it the cumulative result of twentieth-century progress? The controversy goes on, and meanwhile thousands of people suffer from devastating physical exhaustion, pain and bizarre brain symptoms, sometimes for years.

This book is for people who develop ME; for their friends and relatives who have the difficult task of caring for them while not understanding the illness; for family doctors and other health workers; and for anyone else who is interested. It is written by a doctor whose own career was drastically changed by ME and who believes the answer lies in the person, rather than just medicine.

The book brings together everything that is currently known about ME, summarizes the history of outbreaks, and describes recent research. It offers guidelines for self-management and information about various tried therapies. There are sections on nutrition, vitamins and other supplements, mental problems, relationship problems, and advice for carers.

The author gives encouragement by showing that life with ME *can* be fulfilled, if one moves the goal posts of ambitions a lot closer. There are many people with ME who get better, and those who do not can enrich their lives by a revaluation of priorities. This comprehensive evaluation of ME supplies reassurance and information to newly diagnosed ME patients.

ME

Post Viral Fatigue Syndrome

How To Live With It

Dr Anne Macintyre

UNWIN PAPERBACKS
London Sydney Wellington

First published in Great Britain by Unwin ® Paperbacks, an imprint of Unwin Hyman Limited, in 1989.

Unwin Hyman Limited
15–17 Broadwick Street
London W1V 1FP

Allen & Unwin Australia Pty Ltd
8 Napier Street, North Sydney, NSW 2060, Australia

Allen & Unwin New Zealand Pty Ltd with the Port Nicholson Press
Compusales Building, 75 Ghuznee Street, Wellington, New Zealand

---

British Library Cataloguing in Publication Data

Macintyre, Anne, *1953–*
ME, post-viral fatigue syndrome.
1. Man. Myalgic encephalomyelitis
I. Title
616.813
ISBN 0-04-440318-6

Typeset by Computape (Pickering) Ltd, North Yorkshire
Printed and bound in Great Britain by
Cox & Wyman Ltd, Reading

Contents

Preface

A mysterious illness, seemingly never fatal but often making life scarcely worth living, is widespread today. Amongst the thirty to forty names which it is given, myalgic encephalomyelitis (ME) or post viral fatigue syndrome (PVFS) are those best known. Many doctors do not even believe in it.

The plight of sufferers under these conditions is readily understood especially since in its milder and indeed in its more severe forms, it is common for no signs to be found even on specialist examination. Nevertheless the patient may be exhausted and incapable of concentration to the point of being quite unable to undertake even the simplest tasks.

Dr Macintyre (who as a medical doctor belongs to a group especially prone to this infection) gives an excellent and up-to-date account of the features of the disease together with what is known of its 'scientific' background. The 'neurotic' or 'psychiatric' label attached to sufferers is gradually being changed to one of *organic* disease of the nervous and muscular systems, in every bit the same way as pneumonia is an organic disease of the lung.

In addition to tests carried out in this laboratory, evidence is now accumulating, both in Oxford and the United States, indicating biochemical malfunctioning of muscles and real destruction of small regions in the brain. The first step in dealing with this condition is recognition that it really *is* a disease, as real as multiple sclerosis (with which on occasion it could be confused) or muscular dystrophy. In aiding this step Dr Macintyre has written an excellent text, easy to understand, and worthy of attention not only by the lay public but by the Department of Health, whose concern it ought to be. In many ways the illness is similar to AIDS, and though it is never fatal, it deserves the same attention.

Dr Macintyre's book is recommended wholeheartedly; and if, from time to time, treatments are discussed which have not yet undergone stringent trials, then any fault lies with the Department of Health, which has not funded proper research. Sympathy must lie with sick people who clutch at anything in face of the poverty of help they are offered.

E. J. Field, Professor Emeritus, MD, MS, PhD, FRCP
Naomi Bramson Medical Research Trust

Foreword

CLARE FRANCIS

To have ME is to experience hell twice over, firstly through the devastation of the disease itself, and secondly through the lack of diagnosis, information and support that most sufferers are still having to endure.

In the early days of my illness I dragged myself to the local library and combed the medical reference books for some indication of the name and possible causes of this ghastly affliction. I found nothing. My doctor and the various specialists I saw were hardly more helpful. I was eventually told it was a 'virus' – a vague-sounding diagnosis if ever there was one – and that was it. I was given no advice excepting 'total rest', and was offered none of the support which I so desperately needed. On the contrary, I, like so many sufferers before me, was made to feel guilty for my illness, as if I had brought it upon myself. The horrific mental symptoms were put down to reactive depression: had I had an upset recently? An unhappy love affair perhaps? As a single parent, wasn't life a bit much for me? The fact that, until my illness, my life had never been happier or more fulfilled was overlooked. My real mistake, of course, was to have developed an illness which cannot be diagnosed by simple blood tests, which has a bewildering array of strange and sometimes vague symptoms, and for which there is no magic cure.

By the time I had completed the first round of doctors my isolation was almost complete. Not surprisingly, family and friends found it difficult to understand a disease which had no name, no visible symptoms, makes you come apart mentally, yet often leaves you looking perfectly well. Rather than test their loyalty beyond reasonable bounds, I pretended my illness wasn't happening. I covered up the gaping holes in my life with lies and evasions: while I slept all day my answering machine said I was out; when I stumbled over words or walked into things I joked about having had a late night; and my social life was reduced to almost nothing by constantly pleading a previous engagement.

I began to live the life of a recluse – a lonely, isolated and desperate recluse. Looking back, it was a living nightmare. Yet many sufferers have experienced far, far worse: alienation, denigration, loss of employment and the break-up of relationships.

It is my ambition and that of my colleagues in the ME Action Campaign that ME sufferers should never again have to endure their illness in such appalling isolation and ignorance. Although much progress has been made in the recognition of the disease, there is still a very long way to go. In particular, there is an urgent need to reach the many sufferers who, though desperate for information and support, still do not know where to turn.

This book should do much to help those people. It provides the widest and most detailed information on ME yet published. Anne Macintyre, who is both a doctor and a sufferer, has explained the disease in the light of the latest available research, and taken an impartial look at all the various therapies and treatments currently in use.

I hope this book will prevent sufferers from making

the mistakes that I and so many other desperate people have made. I wasted much energy, not to mention money, on traipsing up and down Harley Street seeing numerous doctors, both orthodox and alternative, who swore they knew exactly what was wrong with me (their diagnoses nearly always differed), who pressed me into following their ineffective, bizarre, even dangerous remedies, and who, in the end, left me worse off both physically and financially.

None of the treatments and therapies discussed in this book will effect a miracle cure, for none exists, but all have been tried by ME sufferers and in some cases, though inevitably not all, provided improvement or relief. All of us who have battled with ME over any length of time know the importance of approaching the disease from many different angles simultaneously – diet, supplementation, and lifestyle – and of experimenting to find out what suits us as individuals. This book provides the information on which to build a programme to suit yourself and your unique set of difficulties and problems. Self-help, as most ME sufferers learn through long and hard experience, is the only way forward.

It is unfortunate that sufferers of such a debilitating disease should be thrown back on their own resources, and yet, since self-help is by far the best way of tackling the illness, it is no bad thing. We expect too much of medicine and science. Indeed, we are the victims as well as the beneficiaries of this scientific age. We find ourselves in a situation where, if routine tests cannot pick up an illness, it cannot exist. Textbooks are consulted as if they were written in stone. The medical profession feels bound to give answers even where there are none.

Yet leading scientists will always be the first to

admit that what is known is always exceeded by what is unknown. It is sometimes forgotten that the intricacies of the immune system are only now beginning to be unravelled. And in the field of enteroviruses, which are heavily implicated in ME, virtually all work ceased after the development of the polio vaccine in 1954. Research does not continue in a smooth curve, but in fits and starts instigated by necessity.

Other diseases have had to battle for recognition – notably multiple sclerosis, an illness which also responds to self-help. And other diseases have been misunderstood – isolated cases of polio were often labelled neurotic or hysteric in origin. All became accepted in time.

But however slow acceptance may be in coming, there is the consolation that the majority of ME sufferers do eventually recover. This may offer small comfort to those in the thick of the illness who can see nothing but months of gloom ahead, and for those who have already endured years of unremitting symptoms, but the facts do point to eventual improvement for most.

I have had enormous ups and downs, but experimentation with many of the treatments and remedies described here has brought slow improvement and ever-quicker recovery from relapse. Furthermore, the more I have learnt about the illness, the more I have been able to come to grips with it.

I hope that, for all the sufferers who read this book, it brings a glimmer of light to the end of the tunnel.

List of Abbreviations

ACE	Advisory Centre for Education
ACTH	adrenocorticotropic hormone
AIDS	acquired immune dysfunction syndrome
AK	applied kinesiology
ARMS	Action for Research into Multiple Sclerosis
CFIDS	chronic fatigue and immune deficiency syndrome
CFS	chronic fatigue syndrome
DGLA	dihomo-gamma-linoleic acid
DNA	desoxyribonucleic acid
EB virus	Epstein Barr virus
ECG	electro-cardiogram
EEG	electro-encephalogram
EFAs	essential fatty acids
EMG	electromyography
EPA	eicosapentanoeic acid
EPD	enzyme potentiated desensitization
GABA	gamma-amino-butyric acid
GLA	gamma-linoleic acid
HBLV	human B-cell lymphotropic virus
HHV	human herpes virus
IgA, IGM, etc	immuno globulins
MAOIS	mono-amine-oxidase inhibitors
ME	myalgic encephalomyelitis
MEAC	ME Action Campaign
MRI	magnetic resonance imaging

MS	multiple sclerosis
MSC	Manpower Services Commission
NHS	National Health Service
NI	National Insurance
NK lymphocytes	natural killer
NMR	nuclear magnetic resonance
PABA	para amino benzoic acid
PG	prostaglandin
PVFS	post viral fatigue syndrome
RDA	recommended daily allowance
RNA	ribonucleic acid
TM	transcendental meditation
VDUs	visual display units
VPI	virus protein I

Introduction

There are at least 150,000 people in Britain today who are suffering from a strange illness which nobody yet understands. This illness can have a devastating effect on one's life.

My own story is a typical example. Five years ago I was able to work full time in a busy hospital department, and to spend my free time gardening, decorating an old house, socializing and generally living a full life. I went to Scotland every year, and was able to achieve a whole day's hill walking, maybe 18 miles. Like most people, I got colds in winter, and sometimes felt worn out after a busy day.

Four years ago, during a spell of very hard work while in India, I had a severe throat infection, but had to carry on working. After I returned home I remained unwell and tired for many weeks. Over the following three years I had periods of severe exhaustion alternating with short spells of nearly normal energy. My doctor could find nothing wrong, and did lots of tests which were all normal.

I had bouts of unexplained depression and feelings of utter 'awfulness', when I felt more ill than at any previous time in my life. I had to cut down my work to part time, and to rest when not working. In the past I had found that a long walk in the countryside, or a swim, would lift me out of 'the blues'. But now, any exercise was having a disastrous effect, and I had more benefit from spending the weekend just sitting in a chair. I knew that something was wrong, but no one could identify it. I feared that I was very neurotic or maybe losing my mind.

Then a flu-like illness in August 1987, which featured fever and terrible muscle pains, seemed to plunge me into a worse state. Over the following three months, I became unable to walk 50 yards without collapsing, my brain turned into cotton wool, I was unable to read or bear the sound of music, weird symptoms plagued me, including waking in the night with palpitations and loud noises in my head, my vision was often blurred, I smelt things that were not there. But the overriding problem was the extreme exhaustion brought on by the simplest task, even brushing my hair, or chopping some vegetables.

But I am luckier than many sufferers. I found out in October 1987 from a physician that I had myalgic encephalomyelitis, and that it had probably started four years ago, with a severe relapse in August. I now know where I stand, and have been enabled to reorganize my life to try to cope with it. My condition has improved a little, now that I have stopped worrying about what is wrong. I have to be very careful not to do too much, not to work in the garden or to try and walk far even on a lovely day. I have not sold my mountain boots, I hope to use them again one day!

This disease has been described all over the world, principally in developed countries. In Britain it was known as Royal Free disease (following an outbreak in 1955 in the London hospital of that name) and also as Iceland disease (where there was an outbreak in 1948–9). A rough estimate of the incidence at present is about 1 in 1,000 people. This makes it as prevalent as Parkinson's disease and more common than multiple sclerosis. In countries where it does not appear to exist, this is because it is not yet recognized by the medical profession, and sufferers are given other labels. In Britain, Canada, Australia and New Zealand, the illness is known as myalgic encephalomyelitis, and in the United States as chronic fatigue syndrome. In this book I shall refer to it as ME.

I decided to write this book to provide useful information for people who think they may have ME and want to find out; for those who have been told they are suffering from it, but that there is no treatment; for friends and relations of sufferers; and for any doctors who still do not believe that ME is a genuine disease.

Many sufferers cannot obtain any diagnosis from their doctors and, even worse, some are labelled neurotic or hysterical after doing the rounds of various specialists. It is a sad fact of twentieth-century medicine that a diagnosis of disease depends more on laboratory tests and X-rays than on careful history-taking and examination. ME is a diagnosis based on the history of the patient's illness, and to date there is no single diagnostic test which gives a 100 per cent accurate answer.

The only branch of medicine that does not depend on tests or abnormal physical findings is psychiatry, and it is into this pigeon-hole that many ME patients are put. I wonder how many people are languishing in mental institutions who would be relieved to be told that they have a recognized organic disease, and whose health could improve from a regime that does not consist only of psychotropic drugs? This does not deny that very many people with ME do have mental symptoms as part of their disease.

Getting a diagnosis is one thing, and what a relief it is to know what is wrong with you. The next problem is: where do I get advice? Is there any cure? Is there anything that I can do for myself to improve things? The answer to this last question is **yes**, and people with ME will cope a lot better if they stop expecting medical science to provide a cure, and instead they set about organizing their own plan of action – or rather their plan of **in-action**; recovery from ME requires much less activity and more rest. One needs to learn to give more time to simply **being** and less to **doing**.

If you who start to read this book have ME, then the chances are that you find it hard to concentrate for long. If you decide that you have read enough for today, please remember just two things:

(1) You can certainly improve and have a good chance of some recovery.
(2) The more you rest now and stop trying to achieve anything, the less frustrated you will be by your limitations, and the better your chances of improving.

We live in a culture which worships achievement and all that goes with it. I can offer no proof, nor scientific explanation, that ME is a disease of the twentieth century and of 'developed' nations. But since the illness is made worse by both physical and mental effort, I wonder how prevalent it is in communities which practise meditation, prayer and tranquillity – such as a Buddhist monastery?

There is no doubt that ME follows on from a viral infection in most sufferers, whether the infection is noticed or not. But surely there must be other factors involved? For why, in a family or group who all contract the virus, does only one person go on to develop ME? At the time of writing, there is no answer to this. Something must be happening to the immune systems of these people that is allowing the illness to develop.

I see no reason for people who have this illness to wait until it has been fully explained, before having some information and ideas about self-help.

This book brings together everything that is known so far about ME, and all known ways of coping with it. Some ways are based on my own experience, others I have gleaned from other sufferers. There is nothing offered in the way of self-management which is harmful, even though some methods have not yet been proven by controlled medical trials. One problem in testing treatments for ME is the up-and-down course of the illness, which makes any improvement difficult to evaluate. But we cannot wait for ever for permission to try and get better ourselves.

The Chinese have used acupuncture for thousands of years, because they observed that it worked. They have not been troubled by the fact that no-one has discovered exactly *how* it works; therefore if something seems to be helpful for a person with ME it is sensible to pass on the information to others.

What is beneficial to one sufferer may not help another. However, **rest** is universally essential. Each person should learn to listen to his or her own body, and co-operate with it to help recovery.

I hope that this book will be helpful for sufferers with ME, and those who care for them. I hope it can give encouragement to anyone who has been compelled by this illness to come to a halt in a busy life, and who may be baffled and depressed by the experience. I have written from the viewpoint of a sufferer, and also as a doctor.

In recent years there has been a lot of valuable research into ME; the threads of understanding are starting to be woven together to make a picture of the disease process. More research projects are being planned, and several treatments are going to be tested in the USA. We can look forward to a time when the mystery of this devastating illness is solved, and hope that some definitive cure will become available.

1
What is ME?

It has various names, this disease which causes profound exhaustion, pain, and mental confusion, and which leaves so much disability and suffering.

Some of these names are:

- Yuppie disease – because it is thought to strike people who are high achievers
- Chronic Epstein Barr virus – in USA
- Chronic fatigue syndrome – in USA
- Icelandic disease – from an outbreak in Iceland
- Tapanui flu – from an outbreak in New Zealand
- Epidemic neuromyesthenia
- Royal Free disease – from the 1955 London epidemic.
- Post viral fatigue syndrome

Whatever it is called, it is a very unpleasant condition. The main symptom is **profound exhaustion**, mental and physical, **made worse by exercise**, with a variety of other bizarre symptoms, in a person who may look well, and in whom there are virtually no abnormal signs on examination.

The effects of this disease can be devastating to someone who was previously active and led a full life. Not only are jobs lost and early retirement made necessary for many, but marriages may founder, relationships and friends be lost, and many hobbies and interests dropped. Even the most basic tasks of daily living may require such herculean effort that the sufferer cannot survive without help. Some ME sufferers are prisoners in their bodies, and so the condition has been referred to by some as 'a living death'.

Added to all this suffering is the fact that for decades, the disease was not recognized by the medical profession, apart from a few perceptive doctors, and patients were labelled as malingerers, neurotic or mad.

Not surprisingly, a few who suffered from this condition have taken their own lives. They were not only very ill, but were denied the basic recognition of their illness and proper medical support.

Myalgic encephalomyelitis is the name which in fact describes the main symptoms:

myalgia = muscle pain
encephalitis = affecting the brain
myelitis = affecting the nerves.

ME is not as simple as the name implies. It is not one single disease with a course of events and a clearly understood cause, such as we see in chickenpox, for example. To be more accurate, one should call it the 'ME syndrome'; a syndrome means a collection of symptoms which, put together,make a recognizable disease picture, and may be the common end-point of a number of different causes.

ME is recognized in a patient with these features:

(1) Gross, abnormal *muscle fatigue*, which occurs after a relatively small effort, and from which the patient may take days to recover. This is quite unlike any fatigue ever experienced before.
(3) A variety of neurological (encephalitic) symptoms, most prominent being loss of ability to concentrate, impaired memory and disturbances of sensation.

(3) Unpredictable variation in severity of symptoms from week to week, day to day, even hour by hour.
(4) A tendency to become chronic over many months or years.

Everyone feels tired when he or she has a bout of influenza, a cold or any infection. Most people who get a severe dose of influenza will be slightly under par for weeks, possibly months. Glandular fever and hepatitis are well known for the debility which persists for months. These conditions of prolonged recovery are accurately called 'post viral fatigue states'. However, the diagnosis of ME should probably not be made unless the patient has the characteristic features mentioned above.

Most of the advice given in this book is quite appropriate for people who are suffering a post viral fatigue state, whether or not they are going to be labelled as ME, the distinction between ME and other post viral syndromes being one of chronicity, severity and certain symptoms; in a number of patients it is not clear which category they come under.

Many doctors say they find ME hard to diagnose, or to distinguish from a state of chronic depression. Sadly, many doctors still label the patient as malingering or hysterical. However, for most GPs, it is a condition 'once seen, never forgotten'.

In homeopathic medicine, where ME and other post viral syndromes have long been recognized, it is called the 'never well since I had such and such' illness.

ME usually follows on from an infection of some kind, usually some flu with sore throat, glands in the neck, fever, often muscle aching in neck or chest muscles, maybe vomiting and diarrhoea (gastric flu).

There may be a period of apparent recovery, lasting a few weeks; this is followed by inexplicable symptoms coming on, such as sudden collapse, vertigo, severe chest pains, apparent recurrence of the flu or abdominal symptoms. At this stage, no one knows what is going on, and the patient may be put on antibiotics, sent to a cardiologist or other appropriate specialist and given a few weeks off work. 'You've not got over that bug that you had last month, another fortnight of rest should sort it out.' Complete rest for several weeks at this stage may lead to recovery.

But most people expect to be back to normal a few weeks after an infection. And so the patient struggles back to work or school when the expected time limit for recovery expires; then follow months of exhaustion, of inability to perform life's daily tasks, a struggle to keep going, believing that 'mind over matter' will win – and it doesn't; the patient's symptoms get worse, he or she may be very depressed or even suicidal. The patient cannot believe that this pathetic creature whose muscles don't work, whose brain is like porridge, who cries from pain and exhaustion from doing nearly nothing – maybe just trying to get upstairs – can ever be the same fit and active individual he or she was before.

And it is now realized that battling on and trying to become some sort of normally functioning person, is the *worst possible thing to do*. This is why it is so crucial that people know about the existence of ME, because if complete rest is allowed early on, before the full picture develops and it becomes chronic, then there is a chance of early recovery.

Unfortunately, most people expect a cure for nearly every ill nowadays. Old-fashioned principles of allowing the body to heal with rest, good food, fresh air and tranquillity, have been forgotten; the majority of people only allow one or two weeks to recover from a viral infection. If you had tuberculosis, or double pneumonia, or rheumatic fever, would you expect to be back working full tilt after one or two weeks? – of course not. It appears that one common mechanism which triggers off the development of ME is getting a viral infection while one is exhausted or highly stressed, and not resting enough.

However, some sufferers cannot pinpoint the onset of their illness, and have gradually become more tired and ill over a period of time. On careful questioning, though, a history of an infection some time around the date of 'when were you last well?' will be remembered. The triggering infection may have seemed innocuous at the time. It is easy to remember an attack of influenza; however one of the commonest viruses now implicated in ME is the group called 'enteroviruses', which may give a day or two of mild diarrhoea called 'summer flu', and be overlooked.

Most of the earlier observations about ME have been based on patients studied during epidemics. In fact ME occurs in both epidemic and endemic (isolated cases) form, and obviously a cluster of cases in one area will attract more attention than single, apparently unconnected, cases scattered about. There is a history of recorded outbreaks going back to 1934, when an epidemic of what at first seemed to be poliomyelitis was reported in Los Angeles. Since then there have been no less than fifty-two recorded outbreaks in various parts of the world.

The Los Angeles epidemic had features which initially resembled poliomyelitis. At the Los Angeles County General Hospital, 198 staff became ill. The main features which differed from polio were:

(a) Severe muscle wasting, as would be expected in polio, did not occur.
(b) Muscle pain and tenderness, plus sensory symptoms, lasted longer.
(c) Memory lapses, loss of concentration, sleep disturbances, emotional instability, and inability to walk a short distance without fatigue were common symptoms.
(d) Over 50 per cent of the staff were still unable to work six months after the peak of the epidemic.

The best known outbreak of ME in Britain took place in 1955, when nearly 300 members of hospital staff at London's Royal Free Hospital developed what was obviously an infectious illness, over a period of 4½ months. Of these ill members of staff, 255 had to be admitted to hospital; yet only 12 of the patients who were already in the hospital during the epidemic developed the disease. It is probable that the patients were protected from developing the muscle and neurological symptoms of ME because they were resting in bed, whereas the hospital staff were busy and physically active when they became infected. In this way, ME behaves like polio in an epidemic.

The clinical features of this epidemic among Royal Free Hospital staff (doctors, nurses, ancillary and administrative) were as follows:

(1) Malaise, headache, sore throat, abdominal pain, maybe diarrhoea, nausea, enlarged glands. These were the initial symptoms and they fluctuated for several days.
(2) Severe pain in the back, neck or limbs, or in rib margins, and dizziness, sometimes true vertigo. These symptoms came on after a few days.
(3) Neurological signs and symptoms, developed

> usually by the third or fourth week. Seventy-four per cent of patients showed evidence of involvement of the central nervous system. Symptoms included double vision, difficulty in swallowing, paralysis of the face, weakness of arms and legs, twitching or spasms of muscles, and bladder difficulties.
>
> Spontaneous pain, usually with muscle tenderness in weak limbs, was a common feature.

There are some among the staff who were ill, who still suffer today from the illness, which was called epidemic neuromyesthenia. The infectious agent responsible was not isolated.

A full account of the many outbreaks since 1934 has been written by Dr Melvin Ramsay, in his book *The Saga of Royal Free Disease*.

The outbreak in Iceland in 1948–9 is very interesting because in 1955 there was a poliomyelitis epidemic on the island which did not produce cases in the districts where the epidemic neuromyesthenia had occurred in 1948. This implied that whatever virus was responsible for the ME provided protection against polio.

The clinical features of the many outbreaks worldwide (for example, Los Angeles 1934, Iceland and Adelaide 1949–51, Coventry 1953 and Durban 1955, which all corresponded with epidemics of poliomyelitis) had certain features in common:

- An obvious infection
- Involvement of the central nervous system
- Prolonged fluctuating course
- Marked muscle fatigability
- Exhaustion
- A proportion of patients left with many years of physical incapacity.

Case History

The following account is a typical history of an isolated case, and illustrates the importance of diagnosis.

STORY OF MRS J.M.

Jean is a dentist, and married with two teenage sons. She was 41 when she had a bout of diarrhoea following a meal out at a hotel.

> I didn't seem to recover from that, I felt very weak. I was very overworked, looking after sick and elderly grandparents. This was about five years ago. I'd had a hysterectomy a year previously, which was followed by various complications, and I'd had a very nasty bout of flu before the hysterectomy.
>
> After the diarrhoeal illness my energy levels went down and up, and I would get attacks of flu, and low grade fever, with tremendous exhaustion and weakness, lasting for several days.
>
> It was over a year before I was sent to hospital for tests. During this time my main symptoms were complete and utter exhaustion, severe aching muscle pains, inability to concentrate, inability to function normally – I was trying to run a job and a family. My ears became very irritated and painful from sound. I got very depressed, and iller and iller, and was more or less bedridden for about two years. I could just about get out to shops and back, then collapsed in bed. I had to give up my job.
>
> I developed allergies to various foods which had not upset me previously. After I had become more and more ill for over a year following the tummy bug, my GP referred me to an infectious diseases unit for tests. I had various blood tests, and the consultant thought I had a Coxsackie virus. He

heard my story and told me I was ill with myalgic encephalomyelitis, and that he did not know how to make me better. I was too ill at the time to take much in, but at least, knowing I was ill, I could rest.

The rest has been the main cure. Over two years I was so weak that all I could do was get out of bed and collect the things to prepare a meal and take them back to bed. I found cutting a carrot hard work. If I put coal on the fire, that took so much energy I had to go back to bed again. I had great difficulty sleeping for two years, because of the pain. I had two admissions to a psychiatric unit because of severe depression. Sometimes I was so tired that it was an effort to breathe. Once when I felt very ill, my temperature went very low for a few weeks.

It was about a year after I got a diagnosis before I started to get better. My improvement has not been steady – the relapses always occur after physical effort. Once, when I was a bit better, I had to stand in queues at a hospital clinic with a grandparent whom I was accompanying, then foolishly had to push the car which wouldn't start, to take her home. I thought, with the adrenaline of the moment, that I could do it! I came home, collapsed into bed, and I could not get up for a month. My brain packed in, I couldn't function, and it took me months to get over it.

Last year I began to get a bit better. My GP thought that a little physiotherapy would do me good because I was so weak. It was disastrous, even hydrotherapy, although I felt great for the first week, but after 10 days the aching and slight fever came back.

When I was very ill I had dreadful ulcers in my mouth, and Fungilin lozenges helped enormously. It was thought to be a candida infection.

I am now on a total 'no exercise' campaign. As

long as I lie or sit, I can function mentally. Even at my worst, I tried to put clothes on every day, this kept the circulation going, and provided enough exercise to stop me seizing up.

I found that complete bed rest when the temperature was up was beneficial, but only for a short time; when the temperature had settled I tried to get dressed every day.

The first year of the illness I kept fighting it, so of course I just got worse. To begin with it was physical exhaustion. In the second year, I found the mental problems got worse. I couldn't finish a sentence I had started, and my brain switched off. It was so frustrating, I just wept. I felt completely useless, I was just a burden to everybody. I used to say to the boys, 'Put me out for the dustmen in a black plastic bag'!

Jean is now in the fifth year of the illness, but is slowly and steadily getting better. She works one half-day a week, and is able to go out some evenings with her family. The food allergies have improved, but she finds that sticking to a wholefood diet with plenty of salads, not a lot of meat, and no bread, sugar or cakes, helps her. A large meat meal robs her of energy.

Her husband and children were very supportive. 'He got me better through the emotional side of it. When you are very ill, you need lots of love and support. The members of my church have been very helpful, and I had several healing sessions.'

Findings of a Recent Survey

In a recent questionnaire survey (one of several) of people who thought they had ME, of those who gave a fairly typical history and had the cardinal symptoms, 30 per cent had still *not* been recognized as ME by their GPs or consultants.

Symptoms

The following were the various symptoms given, roughly in order of frequency:

- *Made worse by exercise* 100%
- Exhaustion 85%
- Muscle weakness
- Muscle pain – commonest in back of shoulders, upper arms and thighs
- 'Feeling awful' – not a recognized symptom medically!
- Blurring of vision, sometimes actual double vision
- Pins and needles or numbness
- Loss of concentration
- Abdominal swelling
- Headache
- Difficulty in speech – e.g. wrong word, or cannot find the word
- Poor circulation – cold hands and feet
- Pain in the back of the neck
- Abnormal sweating – often with a sour smell
- Dizziness or feeling faint
- Impairment of memory, especially for recent events
- Breathing difficulty
- Sensitive to sound – called 'hyperacusis'
- Noises in ears – called 'tinnitus'
- Sleep disturbance
- Palpitations, and/or racing heart beat
- Difficulty in standing – classic symptom of ME
- Vivid or bad dream

- Joint pains – which may move from joint to joint
- Feeling 'spaced out', disorientation
- Depression
- Loss of sexual interest
- Nausea
- Trembling or shaking
- Chest pains
- Emotional lability – crying easily, rapid mood change
- Constipation
- Recurrent sore throats
- Lymph glands enlarged or painful
- Diarrhoea
- Increased sense of smell
- Altered sense of taste – often 'metallic'
- Twitching muscles
- Abdominal pain
- Vertigo
- Difficulty with balance
- Difficulty in walking, or limited to very short distance
- Back pain
- Panic attacks
- Poor temperature control
- Poor co-ordination – clumsiness
- Pallor when ill – quite common
- Poor bladder control
- Sneezing – as in hay fever
- Pain in face
- Skin very sensitive to touch
- Spontaneous bruising
- Strange skin rashes
- Thirst
- Difficulty in swallowing.

These symptoms are not present all of the time, but the features common to most are *exhaustion* and *symp-*

toms worse for exercise. Most patients said that both mental and physical exhaustion can result from either physical exercise *or* mental effort.

All women who menstruated said that their symptoms worsened before and during a period.

Age and sex distribution

Male : Female	1 : 3
Age	%
under 20	3.5
20–29	15
30–39	28.5
40–49	23
50–59	20
over 60	10

Duration of illness – at time of response (%)

Less than 2 years	35
over 2 years	65
over 5 years	33
over 10 years	12
over 20 years	4

Various other studies have produced slightly different figures, but it seems that, from the date of onset of the illness, one has about a 25–30 per cent chance of still having some symptoms of ME after five years. Of course many of the chronic sufferers may not be as badly afflicted after five years as they were at the outset. Also, most will not have been continuously ill, but will have had remissions and relapses.

Another way of predicting the future is this:

If you are in the first year of the illness, the chances of getting better are

50% in 2 years
60% in 5 years
and 90% in 10 years.

A long list of symptoms has been given. Most of them occur in many other diseases and are non-specific. So what are the features which are most suggestive of ME?

Summary of Typical ME Symptoms

(1) *History of a virus infection* before onset.
(2) *Exhaustion* which is totally out of proportion to the effort made.
(3) *Symptoms which suggest a chronic or recurrent infection*: Low-grade fever; tender lymph nodes; sore throat.
(4) *Muscle problems*: Muscle weakness brought on after minimal effort, which can take several days to improve; Inability to stand – the patient's legs shake and ache after standing for a short time, he or she has to sit down; Cannot hold arms up – e.g. cannot hang up washing; Difficulty carrying bags or even saucepans; Aching back or neck if sitting in unsupporting chair; Intermittent blurring of vision – due to fatigue of ciliary (focusing) eye muscle, or to fatigue of muscles which control eye movements to maintain a single image; Cannot hold a telephone receiver; Aching in face after speaking or chewing; Cannot write a long letter; Muscle tenderness, with very sensitive local spots.

Note that problems arise from *sustained* muscle use; the muscle function may be normal to start with, but pain/aching and fatigue set in after a short time. Slow walking may be easier than standing. The muscles commonly affected are the 'girdle' muscles – back of shoulder, buttocks and thigh.

(5) *Encephalitic, or brain symptoms*: Hypersensitive to sound – may be so severe that voices, radio, ticking clock, are all unbearable; Altered sensation – e.g. clothes hurt if they touch skin, numbness, creepy-crawly feelings; Increased sense of smell, or bizarre smells; Poor concentration – typically, concentration cannot be sustained without brain fatigue, e.g. radio, reading, or following a conversation; Poor short-term memory – forgetting name of someone you know well, forgetting what has just been said; Nominal asphasia – cannot find the word for something; Speech becoming muddled when tired, even slurred; Nightmares, sleep disturbance.

(6) *Autonomic nervous system* (which controls all involuntary body functions): Sudden racing heart beat, or palpitations; Profuse sweating, even when cold; Pallor – often ashen grey – at onset of feeling ill; Poor temperature regulation – e.g. getting into bed with all clothes on to get warm on a summer day, or feeling hot when everyone else is cold; Poor circulation to hands and feet – e.g. chilblains in June; Alternating diarrhoea and constipation; Attacks of low blood sugar; Difficulty in passing urine, urgency or incontinence.

(7) Sudden mood changes, untypical of the person; Development of new allergies – particularly to chemicals and some foods; Difficulty breathing – especially at night, the 'I wake up feeling I cannot get enough oxygen' symptom.

The natural progression of the illness is a slow improvement, **if proper rest is allowed**. Most sufferers relapse because they are active by nature and, when they start to feel better, they do too much and have a relapse.

Main Causes of Relapse

- *Physical exercise*
- Developing another virus infection
- Emotional stress
- Hormonal changes – e.g. menstruation, and after pregnancy
- Surgery
- Various life stresses – e.g. moving house, marriage, divorce, changing jobs, etc.
- Exposure to chemicals
- Sudden change of climate
- Winter – not only the cold, but lack of daylight
- Dental treatment.

There are a small number of sufferers who do not seem to have any remissions, and who gradually deteriorate, but these are relatively few. More often the illness fluctuates, with relapses and remissions occurring, sometimes quite unpredictably. This is one of the features of ME which makes it so hard to assess clinically, especially in any trial of treatment. The marked variations in symptoms and in the degree of illness felt by a sufferer also leads to disbelief from family, friends and the family doctor. People find it hard to accept that you have a genuine illness if they see you in a wheelchair one week, and walking the next. What they don't see is that you can still only walk a short way, and they don't observe your collapse when you get home!

The Controversy – is ME a Disease, or All in the Mind?

In 1970, two psychiatrists at the Middlesex Hospital, London, produced two papers in the *British Medical Journal*, 'Royal Free epidemic of 1955: a reconsideration', and 'Concept of benign myalgic encephalomyelitis'.

In these papers they gave their reasons for considering that the Royal Free epidemic of 1955 had been an outbreak of mass hysteria, and that other outbreaks in the world also had features of hysteria. They admitted that those outbreaks which showed a resemblance to poliomyelitis probably weren't mass hysteria.

In spite of the fact that there were obvious flaws in their reasoning – such as the high incidence of signs of infection and neurological involvement, which could not be hysterically produced – the 'explanation' of ME given by Dr McEvedy and Dr Beard was seized upon by the media, and has unfortunately been accepted without question by a large number of the medical profession ever since, from 1970 until the present time.

The damage done to people who have had this illness, both those of the Royal Free outbreak and others since, has been incalculable. Of course it is much more convenient for everyone – apart from sufferers – to label the condition as hysterical; there is then no need to organize any research into the illness, patients can be ordered to pull up their socks and go back to work, and those who have no direct experience of the nature of the devastating symptoms can rejoice in being far too well balanced to get 'that sort of complaint'. A great deal of money is saved by not having to pay for research into an imaginary disease, nor to providing sickness benefit for imaginary patients.

However, thanks to the tireless efforts of certain doctors who never doubted the reality of the disease, in the last few years evidence has emerged, through various research studies, of the real and organic nature of the illness. Special credit is due to Dr Melvin Ramsay, who was consultant in infectious diseases at the Royal Free Hospital at the time of the 1955 outbreak, and has devoted a large part of his long life to working for recognition of, and research into ME.

Not only some of the doctors, but also patients themselves have campaigned for better recognition and understanding. The ME Association, founded in 1976, and the recently formed ME Action Campaign, have provided support and information to sufferers and have worked to educate doctors, the social services, and politicians about the nature of the illness and its debilitating effects.

Sadly there has been a backlash from some sections of the media to the heightened interest in ME patients. Just when thousands of ill people were at last beginning to be believed by their families, employers and doctors, a programme about the illness was shown on TV. In the studio 'discussion' the impression was given that very few people going to their doctors with symptoms of crippling exhaustion and inability to function had anything much wrong with them that could not be cured by 'a good night's sleep'. The programme also put across the message that there was no benefit to be had from getting a diagnosis, and so people thinking they might have ME should not bother trying to find out.

And then an article appeared on the front page of a widely read 'quality' Sunday paper, with the headline blazed:

YUPPIE FLU ALL IN THE MIND SAY DOCTORS

In fact the article which followed did not say this; but someone felt sufficiently strongly that it was time to put ME back where it belonged, to use that damaging headline.

It is salutary to note that about 20 years ago, unfortunate victims of that most disabling condition, multiple sclerosis, were labelled as neurotic or hysterical. Now MS is recognized, and yet its diagnosis is largely a clinical one; there is still no single specific test for MS which is widely available.

Case History

In case any of you reading this doubt that the McEvedy and Beard diagnosis is still around, let me relate the account of a mother's difficulty when her daughter became ill:

> My daughter aged 11 fell ill with a virus which was going round her school. She did not recover properly, and for months she kept on having swollen glands, vague sore throat, and a slight fever. She was keen to go to school, but some days she would fade out by mid morning and have to come home. If she did any sports or gym she collapsed. I took her to our GP who did some tests which were all normal. He referred her to a hospital paediatrician, who did more blood tests and found nothing wrong. We then took her to a different children's doctor, privately; he charged us a lot of money, said he could find nothing wrong, and that she should be encouraged to go to school. We took her to see a consultant rheumatologist, because she had these

awful pains in her muscles and legs, and he told us that she just needed to exercise and get fit!

Then I saw an article in the *Telegraph* which described her condition exactly. We were so relieved to find out what was wrong. I went back to see the private specialist and showed him the newspaper article, saying 'Look at this, our daughter has got post viral fatigue syndrome, also called ME'. He just dismissed it, and said 'Oh, that's Royal Free Disease, that's been proven to be hysteria'.

We were upset and angry. I knew she was ill and not putting it on. The trouble was that we needed a doctor to give a diagnosis so that she could rest from school if unwell, and be excused from having to do any sport.

It was at this stage that this worried mother told me this story, and fortunately I was able to put her in touch with a more knowledgeable GP, who recognized the illness with no difficulty. Happily the girl is now gradually improving, and less than a year after having the virus is able to go to school, provided she is careful about exercise.

But there were three specialists, all in one not very large city, who could not recognize that this child was ill, and more importantly did not give the crucial advice that rest was essential.

Terminology – Names of ME

The definition of the 'ME syndrome' has caused doctors problems over the years. In order for the condition to be recognizable, and also to improve the basis for clinical research, a working case definition was required – one which could be accepted worldwide. In the USA, a number of physicians got together and between them they have drawn up the criteria for case definition of *chronic fatigue syndrome* (CFS), the name they have proposed. Another name recently proposed in the USA is chronic fatigue and immune dysfunction syndrome (CFIDS).

At the time of writing, these terms – CFS or CFIDS – have not been adopted by British doctors, but it is worth giving the case definition here, as it is a useful one, and may become internationally recognized.

(a) *Major critiera* – both to be fulfilled:
  (1) *New* onset of persistent or relapsing, debilitating fatigue or easy fatigability in a person with no such previous symptoms, that does not resolve with bed-rest, and is severe enough to reduce daily activity below 50 per cent of what it was before the illness, for at least six months.
  (2) Other clinical conditions which could cause this fatigue must be excluded by history, examination, and appropriate investigations. (Then a long list of such conditions, and the various necessary tests, is given.)

(b) *Minor criteria – symptoms* which must have persisted or recurred over six months, and have developed at or after the onset of fatigue:
  (1) Mild fever or chills
  (2) Sore throat
  (3) Painful lymph glands
  (4) Muscle weakness
  (5) Muscle pain or tenderness
  (6) Prolonged (24 hours or more) fatigue following a level of exercise that previously caused no problems

(7) Headaches different in type to any experienced before the illness
(8) Joint pains
(9) Neuropsychologic complaints (encephalitic) – one or more of the following: light sensitivity, blind spots in vision, loss of memory, irritability, confusion, poor concentration, inability to think clearly, depression
(10) sleep disturbance.

(c) *Physical criteria* – observed by a doctor at least twice, and at least a month apart:
(1) Low grade fever
(2) Inflamed throat
(3) Palpable or tender lymph nodes in neck or armpits.

Eight or more of symptom criteria are needed, or else at least two physical and at least six of the symptoms, in addition to the two major criteria.

In the USA, more emphasis was previously given to chronic Epstein Barr virus as a likely cause than in the UK. This may be why there is such emphasis on fever, sore throat, and tender lymph glands. Many of the ME patients I know of in the UK never have a fever, but rather have subnormal temperatures, and do not have enlarged lymph glands.

Dr A. R. Lloyd of New South Wales, Australia, and colleagues (*Lancet*, June 4 1988) have agreed that the best term is chronic fatigue syndrome. They have developed a set of diagnostic criteria after reviewing 100 patients:

(1) Chronic or relapsing fatigue, made worse by very minor exercise, causing disruption of daily life, and of over six months duration

(2) Neuropsychiatric dysfunction including impairment of concentration, and/or short-term memory loss, and/or
(3) Evidence of abnormal cell mediated immunity.

The following findings, in addition, are supportive:
muscle pain, joint pain, headaches, depression, tinnitus, paraesthesiae (abnormal sensations), sleep disturbance, lymph glands, sore throats.

Dr Lloyd and colleagues consider that the name 'post viral fatigue syndrome' is wrong, since the illness is known to be triggered by other infections as well as viruses – e.g. brucellosis and toxoplasmosis, and also by immunizations – e.g. tetanus, typhoid, influenza, cholera.

These observations, coupled with the laboratory evidence of disordered immune function in many patients, suggest that something is challenging the immune system. Something triggers off the disease, most commonly a viral infection, in a person whose immune system is already damaged in some way. In the USA, some researchers believe that there is a common agent, possibly the newly discovered HBLT virus (see page 36), which affects the immune response and sets the scene for another virus or something else to start ME.

For the rest of this book, the illness will be called ME. In Australia and New Zealand it is at present called ME syndrome, in Italy chronic influenza; and by various sections of the media it is called 'Yuppie flu'.

Chapter 3 endeavours to explain what is the cause of the ME symptoms and what is happening in the body. But it is not as simple as you might believe from press, TV and radio reports. Before this there is a short chapter about the immune system and some medical terms which will recur in the book. You may, however, proceed to Chapter 3 if you already understand the body's immune system, or if you don't feel up to reading about it!

2

The Immune System

This term is used quite often in this book and in many others about health, so here is a simplified description of what the immune system is.

The body is constantly invaded by 'foreign' substances. The immune system is the natural protective mechanism which prevents damage to the body by invaders. Anything which is 'non-self' is recognized as foreign and is normally disposed of or made harmless by a healthy immune system.

The invader may be:

- Microbes–viruses, bacteriae, yeasts
- Parasites – worms, malaria, etc.
- Foreign tissues, e.g. transplants
- Poisons, e.g. chemicals in food, in air or water, smoke, alcohol, drugs, as well as other poisons
- Cancer cells
- Dust, pollens, moulds.

It is the defensive reaction against a potentially harmful thing that produces symptoms. For example, the pain of a boil is not caused by the germs in it, but results from the swelling and increased blood flow to the area. If there was not this local painful reaction, the infection would not be sealed off and attacked, but could spread throughout the body, with serious results. Similarly, the fever and malaise that is a feature of the common cold is not caused by the virus, but by the chemicals produced by the immune system doing battle with the virus. In fact people whose immune system is not efficient may not have much of a fever when they have an infection.

The army which the body has for its defence consists of white blood cells with different divisions, and their weapons are the various substances made by white cells which help them deal with the invaders.

The *white blood cells* are made in the bone marrow. They are much less numerous than red blood cells, which carry oxygen round the body, but are essential to life. The types of white blood cell are:

(1) *Polymorphs* – meaning changing shape – also called granulocytes, because they contain granules which release chemicals which are poisonous to microbes. They are relatively large, and their main job is scavenging. They are highly mobile and rush in large numbers to the site of an injury or an infection. They can engulf a bacterium by changing shape, and inside produce chemicals which digest the germ. They are found in large numbers in pus.

(2) *Macrophages* – large scavengers of dead tissue and foreign particles.

(3) *Lymphocytes* – there are two sorts,
B lymphocytes, matured in the bursal or lymph tissues, and
T lymphocytes, matured in the thymus gland

There are further subdivisions of *T lymphocytes*, often called T cells. There are *helper* cells, which help the B lymphocytes to produce antibodies, and the polymorphs and macrophages to kill or engulf foreign matter. And when a battle with some invader is over, the *suppressor* cells stop the reaction. There are also *natural killer* cells which destroy infected cells. This is a great oversimplification of the functions of the various platoons of lymphocytes; I doubt that many doctors other than immunologists really understand the immune system in depth.

All white blood cells circulate in the blood and in all tissues of the body, on 'patrol' for invaders, and can move to where they are needed.

The *B lymphocytes* produce *antibodies* to microbes and to their toxins. An antibody is specific for the antigen – *antigen* means the thing which has stimulated the lymphocyte to make the antibody. A second exposure to the antigen induces a greater production of antibody to it, because the recipe for that particular antibody is stored on the surface of 'memory' cells – another function of white cells – and on recognition of the antigen, the B lymphocytes are stimulated to make the antibody.

This is how immunization works, and also why one becomes immune to measles after an attack. These antibodies are called *immunoglobulins*. They are very large molecules of protein and are classified into groups, called IgA, IgM, IgG, IgE (I list all these names because you may hear them mentioned in the results of various blood tests).

The T lymphocytes are active against viruses, as well as helping B cells with their work. Viruses can only survive and replicate inside living cells, so T cells have to be able to kill the cells invaded by the virus.

T cells produce various chemicals called *lymphokines*, one of which is *interferon*, which help in the task of killing infected cells. Lymphokines also cause inflammation, and are involved in allergic responses. These white cell reactions that do not need the antibodies made by B cells, but take place using T cells and their chemical weapons, can be called 'cell mediated immunity'. It is the sort of immune reaction used to overcome chronic infections such as TB.

Anything that (a) reduces the number of white cells; (b) reduces their mobility; and (c) weakens their killing ability, will lessen the body's defence against a virus infection.

3

What Causes ME?

Four blind men came across a creature and tried to find out what it was. Each one found a different part of the animal, and examined it carefully.

One said, 'It is a hosepipe' – examining the trunk.

Another said, 'It is like a tree trunk' – feeling a leg.

The third said, 'It is a snake' – he'd found the tail.

The fourth said, 'This is an odd creature, it lives in a very long shell' – he had hold of a tusk.

None of them was able to see the whole animal, which of course was an elephant.

I think that this is about the stage we are at with describing ME. Of course medical researchers are not blind, and much painstaking valuable work has been done, and is still going on. What has been discovered so far?

- Virologists find ME is usually caused by a virus.
- Immunologists find ME is a disordered immune system.
- Clinical ecologists say ME is a condition of multiple food and chemical allergies.
- Psychiatrists decided (many years ago) that ME is a psychiatric illness – i.e. we are mad.
- Neurologists think ME is a disorder of the nervous system.

Various theories and hypotheses have been put forward around the world:

- some believe ME is caused by pesticides;
- some try to associate it with geopathic stress and electromagnetic radiation from power lines;
- another hypothesis is that ME results from toxic conditions in the large bowel caused by Western diet and antibiotics;
- another theory is that the immune system is altered by immunizations or antibiotics.

Recent researchers have been looking at different aspects of ME:

(1) What virus or viruses cause it
(2) What the virus does in the body
(3) Abnormalities of immune function
(4) Why muscles don't work properly
(5) Red blood cells and cell membranes
(6) Central nervous system abnormalities
(7) Follow up of Iceland's ME patients, 40 years on.

(1) Evidence of Virus Infection

The enteroviruses

In a small town on the Hudson River in New York State in the late 1940s, a new virus was isolated from children with a disease that resembled poliomyelitis. The virus was named Coxsackie after the town. It is now known that Coxsackie viruses are members of a group called *enteroviruses*, which live in the human intestine. The polio virus is another sort of enterovirus. Enteroviruses can affect many systems, but have a particular affinity for the *central nervous system* and *muscles*.

In two outbreaks of ME in Scotland in 1983, there were significant numbers of patients who had antibodies to Coxsackie B virus in higher level than in the general population. Then in a further report of patients with symptoms of ME in a Dumbartonshire practice (1984), nearly half had high Coxsackie B antibody levels.

In this same practice, 55 per cent of those with Coxsackie infection were still ill after one year, and high antibody levels persisted in all but two of the patients.

In 1983, further evidence of a Coxsackie B virus causing ill health in the local population was found by Dr Eleanor Bell, a Glasgow virologist. She found that patients admitted to a general medical ward, mostly with chest pains, also had high levels of Coxsackie B antibody.

So it seemed clear that in Scotland the causative agent of several outbreaks of an illness with all the features of ME was a member of the enterovirus family called Coxsackie.

The human enterovirus family comprises about 70 species:

Polio viruses, Coxsackie A and B, echoviruses, sub groups of these and others. There are records of enterovirus diseases dating back in history to 2000 BC.

Now that a polio vaccine has reduced the incidence of paralytic polio, the *non-polio enteroviruses* are becoming more important in causing human disease. History has shown that enteroviruses have a great capacity to start new syndromes and new epidemics.

Enteroviruses are known to cause many different clinical conditions; examples of enteroviral illnesses are:

- Non-specific infection – e.g. 'summer flu', which may lead to ME

- Respiratory infections
- Gastro-enteritis
- Hepatitis
- Meningitis and encephalitis
- Poliomyelitis
- Bornholm disease (severe chest pains are due to involvement of the intercostal muscles between the ribs
- Myocarditis (heart muscle) and pericarditis
- Hand, foot and mouth disease, and other skin conditions
- Conjunctivitis
- Pancreatitis and juvenile onset diabetes
- Myalgic encephalomyelitis.

Enteroviruses are known to affect muscle and nerve particularly. The two main tissues affected in ME are *muscle* and *nerve*. Or one could say that enteroviruses are 'myotropic and neurotropic'. A number of ME patients have heart muscle involvement (myocarditis).

Enteroviruses are spread from the gut via sewage, rivers, estuaries, beaches and agriculture to reinfect humans in drinking water and food. They are easily picked up on beach and water holidays, by hospital workers from bedpans and other equipment, by those who work with young children – who frequently harbour enteroviruses without signs of illness – and by land and water workers. Most enteroviral infections do not cause any obvious illness.

In several outbreaks of ME, patients were initially thought to have polio (e.g. Los Angeles 1934, Iceland 1948), and health authorities thought a polio epidemic had started, until it became clear that the illness, although resembling poliomyelitis, had some different features (see pages 5–6). One aspect in which ME behaved like polio was that those who were most physically active when they contracted the infection were most likely to develop muscle weakness.

New laboratory proof that enteroviruses are present in a sizeable number of ME patients has come from the work of Professor James Mowbray and colleagues at St Mary's Medical School, London. Their findings published in the *Lancet*, January 1988, are summarized here.

It has always been difficult to detect virus in the stools because it has to be separated from antibody first, so a method was devised which would detect enterovirus-group-protein in the blood.

This protein, called VPI polypeptide, is common to all members of the enterovirus family. VPI was detected in the blood of 51 per cent of a group of ME patients. The number of VPI positives was greater in those patients who also had IgM antibody to enteroviruses.

This VPI test, also popularly called 'Professor Mowbray's test', or the enterovirus test, has since been carried out on the blood of many more presumed ME patients, and is positive in about 60 per cent. If positive, it means that there is active virus in the body. The test does not identify which enterovirus it is, because the virus protein is common to all of them.

So does that mean that if your VPI test is negative, the diagnosis is not ME? *No, it does not*.

Of those with a negative VPI test, about half are likely to have persisting or reactivated Epstein Barr virus, the one that causes 'glandular fever'. The rest may have other, undetected persistent viral illnesses, or have ME with no obvious viral cause.

It is worth quoting here some figures from a recent questionnaire survey of ME patients, showing that *a number of things may trigger off the illness*:

Question: Do you have any idea what infection, if any, started your illness?
Answer: (out of 400 questionnaires)

Proven Coxsackie	18	Chickenpox	2
Glandular fever	31	Toxoplasma	2
Influenza	53	Cytomegalovirus	2
Gastro-enteritis	25	Immunizations:	
'A virus'	70	Influenza	2
Shingles	3	Tetanus	1
Tonsillitis	4	Rubella	1
Pneumonia	4	Typhoid/cholera	1

What is interesting is the range of things other than the expected influenza and glandular fever. These numbers are only of those people who *knew* what they had had – they would be different if all 400 had had full investigations.

The Epstein Barr virus

ME was known as chronic Epstein Barr virus disease in the USA until recently, now it is called chronic fatigue syndrome, or CFS. The EB virus is a member of the herpes family, it is a different animal from an enterovirus; they have different kinds of molecules in the part of the virus which carries the codes for replication. Herpes viruses are 'DNA viruses' and enteroviruses are 'RNA viruses', DNA and RNA being the two types of molecules. EB virus is best known for causing glandular fever, correctly known as infectious mononucleosis. It seems to be present in about 20 per cent of people with ME.

Now glandular fever is well known for the prolonged debility that persists for months after the acute infection, but it is not always easy to draw the line between post glandular fever malaise and true ME. Most people have been infected with the EB virus by the age of 30, usually with few symptoms; only in a few is the infection severe enough to cause glandular fever. So if you look for evidence of previous EB infection, you will find it in about 95 per cent of ME patients, regardless of whether this is what has caused their ME.

Testing for active infection with EB virus requires several tests. (These are listed in Appendix B.)

If tests indicate a current or recent EB virus infection in someone with symptoms of ME, what has happened is this: a latent (i.e. hidden) EB virus that has laid dormant in some body cells for many years, has become reactivated, and has turned into an active infection or a persistent one. The EB virus can hide in surface cells of nose, throat, and in some white blood cells (B lymphocytes), for years, usually causing no trouble, until something happens to allow it to flare up.

Professor Mowbray of London, after testing blood samples from ME patients in the UK and from the USA, has found about 20 per cent Epstein Barr virus positive, and about 60 per cent enterovirus positive, the two groups not overlapping.

In New Zealand, Professor J. C. Murdoch of Otago studied 200 patients with ME syndrome and in 19 per cent there was evidence of continuing infection with EB virus.

It is possible that other viruses which appear to cause ME, such as other herpes viruses, enteroviruses and cytomegalovirus, may also have been reactivated, having been latent for years in the body.

A new virus has recently been described as being a possible culprit in the development of ME. It is the human herpes virus type 6 (HHV–6), also known as human B-cell lymphotropic virus (HBLT–V). However, researchers in Sydney, Australia found no difference in incidence of the HHV–6 between ME patients and healthy controls. In London, research showed that by 1 year of age, about 60 per cent of children already had evidence of infection with HHV–6, showing that the virus is very common and acquired early in life. To quote from the Australian researchers: 'HHV–6 is a virus in search of a disease!'

So, as yet, there does not seem to be one single virus causing ME. It is always possible that an undiscovered 'ME virus' exists, and that those we know about are red herrings, but I doubt this to be so.

(2) What the Virus Does in the Body

Further evidence still of the presence of virus material in some patients with ME has come from the work of Dr Len Archard at Charing Cross Hospital, London. He examined muscle biopsies from patients with classical features of ME, and using a special technique, he found enterovirus specific RNA (ribonucleic acid) in 20 out of 96 muscle biopsies. In the remaining 76 specimens and in all muscle biopsies from healthy controls, enterovirus RNA was not found.

The positive result of 20 out of 96 patients (about a fifth), may be an underestimate, because the muscle tissue affected by the virus is patchy, and a biopsy specimen may not always include a sample of muscle that is affected by virus.

It now seems possible, certainly in ME people with enterovirus, that part of the virus is sitting inside muscle cells and is interfering with the power house machinery.

This is indeed a feature of *persistent virus infections,*

which are increasingly recognized as being involved in several chronic illnesses of unknown cause. In acute viral infections which clear up, there is a reaction by the body's defence system; this results in the death of cells that are infected by the virus, and prevents the virus from infecting other cells; therefore the virus, which can only replicate inside a living cell, stops reproducing and dies out.

However certain viruses are known for their ability to survive in the human and cause persistent infection. These include many herpes viruses (such as Epstein Barr, chickenpox, cytomegalovirus, herpes simplex), rubella and measles viruses, and the AIDS virus, hepatitis B, and others.

> Such viruses may not always kill their host cell in which they replicate, and may not generate immune responses that are effective in clearing the virus ... we discuss how *some viruses can cause disease*, not by destroying the cells that they infect, but *by altering the specialized functions of that cell*. It is likely that such disorders involve primarily the immune, nervous, and endocrine systems. (Southern and Oldstone, 'Medical consequences of persistent viral infection', *New England Journal of Medicine*, February 1986)

ME seems to be a persistent virus infection. Other diseases such as diabetes, parkinsonism and schizophrenia will probably turn out to be caused by persistent virus infections.

A common cry from ME patients is that their muscles and brains don't work properly any more! The concept of a virus sitting inside nerve and muscle cells and interfering with their special functions may at first seem a bit far fetched, but becomes believable if you understand the nature of a persistent virus, as outlined above.

Virus is probably affecting the special function of brain cells, and indeed many other body organs. Some endocrine functions *may* be affected, such as the thyroid gland, the adrenal glands (which produce cortisone, adrenaline and noradrenaline, substances of vital importance in the body's reaction to stress, infection, etc.), the pituitary gland, or ovaries. The pancreas seems likely to be involved in many viral infections, and as a result may not be producing enough pancreatic digestive enzymes; this would lead to poor digestion and absorption of food, especially proteins. There is no part of the body that is never affected by a widespread persistent virus infection. This explains the great variety of ME symptoms!

A persistent virus would also continually stimulate some degree of immune response. This response is not great enough to destroy the virus, but has two main effects:

(a) The constant production of *'lymphokines'*, the chemical weapons made by white cells and other cells as part of an immune response. One of these, *interferon*, causes depression, fatigue, muscle pains and flu-like feelings. This was discovered when interferon was tried out to treat patients with chronic liver infection – the patients complained of typical ME relapse symptoms. Many of the other lymphokines have inflammatory properties and could be causing some of the ME symptoms.

(b) The other effect of an abnormal ongoing immune response (to the persistent virus) is *allergic reactions*. It is known that histamine is produced in tissues infected by a virus, and many people seem to develop allergies following a viral illness. Allergy, to almost everything, is a common development with ME (see Chapter 10).

The question whether someone with a persistent virus infection is infectious to those around them is often raised. The viruses present are carried by a large percentage of the population, sometimes in the throat, or in the gut, without causing any ill health. It does not seem that people with ME are any more likely to spread these bugs about than those without ME.

It is estimated that roughly one in four of ME patients has a close relative or work colleague with the illness. In the case of more than one member of a family being affected, there may be factors other than the virus operating, such as inherited predisposition, or some environmental influence in the house or area. Hopefully further research about causative factors will give some answers to these questions.

So, assuming that a variety of viruses, and indeed other infections and even immunizations, trigger off ME, what other factors are involved? Why is it that a number of people in a community can be infected with something – say an enterovirus, which seems the most likely virus where ME occurs in 'outbreaks' – but only a few develop the ME syndrome?

How can we explain the origin of ME in a person with *no* apparent infection at the onset, and maybe with no definite start to the illness? These patients, who report a gradual loss of health and onset of fatigue, and end up with classical ME syndrome, present the greatest challenge for diagnosis and for understanding how their illness came about. It is most likely that one of the main factors which determines whether you get ME is your natural resistance to viruses, i.e. the working of the immune system.

(3) The Immune System and ME

In a very important piece of research, Dr P. O. Behan and colleagues in Glasgow studied 50 patients who had the ME syndrome. The results were published in 1985. The patients all had various investigations performed, including immunological studies. A number of results showed there to be abnormalities in immune functioning. (The following is rather technical, and can be ignored by people who do not understand immunology.)

(1) The function of lymphocytes to make protein was reduced.

(2) The numbers and ratios of different types of T lymphocytes were abnormal, in both acute and chronic cases. The abnormality in chronically ill patients was found to persist throughout two years of retesting. The T-cell abnormalities were these:

Acute cases (ill less than six months)
Reduction in suppressor T_8 lymphocytes
Other T lymphocytes in normal range
Total T lymphocytes reduced.
Chronic cases (ill from six months, up to 22 years)
Reduction in helper T_4 lymphocytes
Other T lymphocytes in normal range
Ratio of T_4:T_8 cells reduced.

(3) Circulating immune complexes were present in a quarter of blood samples.

(4) Autoantibodies (i.e. antibodies to patient's own tissue) to smooth muscle were found in 36 per

cent, and various other autoantibodies in some others.

Researchers in Harvard found a substantial reduction in natural killer (NK) lymphocytes in ME patients, the first time this sort of defect had been found in any disease.

Professor Murdoch of Otago, New Zealand has recently completed a study which demonstrates that patients with ME have reduced T-cell mediated immunity. He believes that viruses may be present because the immune deficiency allows latent infections to become reactivated. What needs investigating are the reasons why the T-cell function has become abnormal in the first place.

Several researchers have found a deficiency of one or more of the sub-classes of IgG immunoglobulins (antibodies) in some patients with ME – mostly, it seemed, in those whose illness was related to a persistent Epstein Barr virus. This is yet another aspect of poor immune function.

Evidence has been found that in ME patients there is a continual high level of interferon being produced in affected tissues. The anticipated high levels of interferon in the blood were not found consistently in ME patients. But a raised amount of a substance that is produced by interferon activity *was* found.

What about those patients whose ME comes on gradually with no precipitating viral infection? The most likely explanation is that they had some earlier viral illness, such as glandular fever or a tummy bug, years ago, which remained quietly somewhere in the body – latent, not causing any immune reaction at all. Then for some reason there was *something which damaged the immune system*, or lowered the body's resistance, and the latent virus came to life and gradually set off the ME syndrome.

Has a viral infection itself altered the immune response? In the USA some doctors believe that a new virus such as the HHV–6 (see pages 35–6; it is also called HBLI) is the single agent which has caused the damage, setting the scene for reactivating latent viruses, or allowing a new infection such as an epidemic enterovirus to set off ME.

Factors which may injure the immune response

(1) Past viral infections such as hepatitis or glandular fever.
(2) Acute stress, such as a severe emotional shock, trauma, accident or assault; or prolonged unrelieved stress – the study of psychoneuroimmunology demonstrates the close relationship between our emotions, the immune and the endocrine systems.
(3) Immunizations – not proven, but suspected by some doctors. In Denmark, researchers have found an association between ill health and the presence of measles virus particles in the body, thought to be resulting from measles immunization, but not proven.
(4) Dietary deficiencies, particularly lack of amino acids, vitamin C, zinc, essential fatty acids, vitamin A, and some B vitamins.
(5) Environmental injury – such as pesticides, ionizing radiation, electromagnetic radiation, chemical pollution of air, water, food and soil.
(6) Toxins from yeast overgrowth or from abnormal bacterial activity in the gut (not proven). See Chapter 9.

Pesticides are worth investigating, not only in connection with ME, but with the apparently increasing incidence of new illnesses which were not seen last century, and which may in part be caused by altered immune function.

DDT first came into use during the 1939–45 war. Its use became widespread in the 1950s and 1960s in America, Britain and other European countries. Although DDT has been superseded by more sophisticated chlorinated hydrocarbons, and by organophosphates, its effects on living creatures are insidious, because it is stored in fats and accumulates, passes through food chains, and affects cell membranes.

The terrible damage to living creatures by indiscriminate use of pesticides is graphically documented in the famous book, *Silent Spring*, by Rachel Carson (Pelican Books), first published in 1962, 26 years ago.

Reports from New Zealand indicate that some ME patients being tested for pesticide levels are giving results higher than expected from the general population; however nothing has yet been published on this.

(4) Studies on the Muscle of ME Patients

The discovery of enterovirus RNA in muscle cells has already been described (see page 36). Dr Archard's work is very exciting, because previous research has demonstrated abnormalities of muscle cell function which would explain the muscle fatigability, weakness and pain of ME patients; but no one had been able to explain what was *causing* muscle cells to behave abnormally.

Researchers have been trying to find out what is happening in the muscles of patients with this disabling fatigue syndrome. The muscle problem is summed up by the statement: 'After walking a few hundred yards, I feel as though I have run a marathon – I am exhausted, feel ill, the muscles hurt and feel like jelly, I cannot move another step and feel collapsed, and the leg muscles ache and are tender to touch for days.'

So researchers looked for evidence of some defect of the energy metabolism in muscle cells.

(a) Dr Jamal performed electrophysiological studies on 40 patients, in Glasgow – these patients were from the group extensively studied by Dr Behan (see page 40). The test was electromyography (EMG) of single muscle fibres, and 75 per cent of patients had an abnormal result. Analysis of the test result suggested that there was something wrong with the *muscle fibre cell membrane*, rather than at the nerve–muscle junction.

(b) Another study, using nuclear magnetic resonance (NMR), has demonstrated excessive early acidosis in exercised muscles of ME patients. (NMR is a sophisticated method for assessing biochemical changes in tissues.)

Muscles of patients were tested while being exercised, and excess lactic acid was produced early during exercise. The conclusion drawn was that there was a defect in the balance between two kinds of energy production. One kind of energy reaction uses glucose and makes lactic acid as a by-product; this is called the glycolytic or anaerobic pathway. The other kind uses mainly oxygen and is called the aerobic pathway.

In ME affected muscle there is too much of the

glycolytic energy method, compared to the oxygen route, and so there is too much lactic acid produced. The excess lactic acid could account for the muscle pain, also for the 'general feeling of awfulness' after exercise.

Examination of pieces of muscle under the electron microscope had already shown a visible abnormality – an increase in size and number of Type II muscle fibres, the ones that use the glycolytic metabolism which releases lactic acid.

(c) Professor Peters of Northwick Park Hospital, London has also looked at ME muscle biopsies. He has found there is a reduction in total RNA protein in muscle cells, *and* that the rate of turnover and repair of muscle protein is significantly reduced and impaired. (Unpublished work.)

(d) At the Biolab physiology and clinical centre in London, Dr Stephen Davies and Dr John Howard have developed a test of muscle function which uses fine heat sensors to record muscle activity. In the muscles of ME patients, the recording of muscle activity is grossly abnormal. The muscle at rest shows continual activity, the contraction is normal, but the relaxation of muscle fibres is slow and jerky. There is an abnormally low level of magnesium in the muscle cells, and movement of chemicals across muscle cell membranes is abnormal.

(5) Red Blood Cell and Cell Membrane Abnormalities

A further finding to suggest that in ME patients there may be a fundamental disorder of *cell membrane func-*

tion has come from the observations of Dr Mukherjee and colleagues in Australia.

They examined red blood cells from seven patients at the time of a clinical relapse. In four cases the red cells showed an abnormal shape, marked in two and less severe in the other two. The other cases and control samples showed normal red cells. Such abnormally shaped red cells had previously only ever been seen in the blood of runners who had just completed a marathon – and ME sufferers in relapse say 'they feel as though they have run a marathon' after minimal exertion!

The peculiar shapes of the red blood cells, roundish instead of disc shaped, could be caused by abnormalities of the red cell wall or outer membrane. The blood cells all appeared normal when retested three weeks later, when the patients felt better, indicating that the abnormality in shape is transient and associated with being in relapse.

It has been suggested that impairment of the circulation may be a factor in ME, and certainly red blood cells which are the wrong shape, i.e. more round than flat, would have difficulty in getting through small capillaries, and therefore there would not be enough oxygen delivered to tissues, and especially to working muscles.

This abnormality of cell membranes, as has now been seen in red cells and muscles, needs further research.

A possible explanation of cell membrane dysfunction has been proposed by Dr Wakefield and Dr Lloyd of Sydney, Australia. Some lymphokines have been shown to alter cell membrane function, and to affect energy metabolism in cells.

As explained earlier, there seems to be a constant production of lymphokines during ME, and as well as producing flu-like symptoms, these chemicals could be interfering with cell function in muscles, red blood cells, and in the brain by their action on cell membranes.

(6) Evidence of Involvement of the Nervous System in ME

It is easier to chop out a piece of muscle to examine than to look at the brain in the living patient. The psychological symptoms, the poor memory and concentration, slurred speech, word blocks, loss of balance, poor co-ordination, etc., are well known to ME sufferers.

No one has found an explanation for these symptoms, although it is postulated that persistent virus infection in parts of the brain and spinal cord is probably interfering with the cells' specialized functions, as happens in muscles. This is difficult to prove, and the mental and neurological symptoms of ME have been variously explained by different doctors as hysterical, due to depression, anxiety or overbreathing.

However, *there is now evidence of organic nerve tissue damage in ME.*

Professor E. P. Field, neurologist at the University of Warwick, finds abnormal signs on careful examination of ME patients. The vibration sense is impaired; this has to be tested on various bony sites, not only at the ankle, and compared to the level felt by the tester. He also finds a positive Romberg test in most patients (a test of balance), and often diminished abdominal reflexes. Special tests of fine eye movements are frequently abnormal. This may be part of the reason why so many sufferers have problems in reading.

Professor Field has developed a test for multiple sclerosis diathesis (i.e. the constitutional tendency to MS); in this test, red blood cells are observed moving in an electric field.

There is one specific result for MS, another result for normal people, and another result for those with organic nervous system damage of any kind (stroke, brain infection, etc.).

The blood of ME patients gives the result of *nervous system damage*. This is not a specific test for ME, but it does show that there is something happening in the brain.

Professor Webb, neurologist at St Thomas's Hospital, London, has been investigating the effects of viruses on mice for some years. The mice are infected with neurotropic viruses, and it is found that the virus causes damage in the part of the brain called the thalamus, and that there are disorders in the brain enzymes as a result.

The thalamus is the sensory telephone exchange and relay station for all incoming messages of sensation, and the hypothalamus next to it has important regulatory functions of body temperature, blood sugar, appetite, sleep, hormones, the autonomic nervous system, mood and emotions. Diseases of the thalamus can result in abnormal sensations, including severe pain. There would seem to be a connection between what is happening in mice, and what is going wrong in ME brains.

In the USA, Dr Anthony Komaroff has been using magnetic resonance scans to look at the brain of ME patients. (This NMR machine was also used to demonstrate excess lactic acid in muscles in the UK; see page 44.)

Characteristic 'white spot' brain lesions have been found in 77 per cent of magnetic resonance imaging scans. The abnormalities are thought to represent tiny areas of inflammation in the brain, such as would result from infection or swelling of brain tissue. However these patients did not show evidence of permanent brain damage, and Dr Komaroff thinks that sufferers should not be too alarmed by these findings, as the white spots are also seen in healthy people, though how commonly is not yet known.

This is an exciting development, as it means that some information may be obtained about changes in function, or about tissue damage, in the central nervous system, using a non-invasive method.

In the UK in 1988, a detailed post-mortem analysis was carried out on the brain of a young person who had committed suicide, and who had had all the classic features of ME. This revealed the presence of virus in part of the brain. Further details are awaiting publication at the present time. It is not possible at the existing stage of research to correlate the post-mortem findings with the 'white spots' found in the US MRI studies.

All these findings do show that something is causing damage in parts of the central nervous system in ME. *However*, the damage may be temporary and not progressive, so do not start to fear that all ME brains gradually seize up, even though there may be times when it feels like it!

(7) The Iceland Research – Akureyi, Forty Years Later

In Iceland in 1948, the outbreak of an illness that resembled polio, but was epidemic myalgic encephalomyelitis, was centred around a small community at Akureyi. A doctor from Canada, Dr Byron M. Hyde, has recently visited Iceland, and was able to study ten people, who are still living, who fell ill during this outbreak. Dr Hyde has consented to his very significant findings being reported here.

Ten people aged between 58 and 84 were interviewed, examined and had blood tests performed. Only two out of the ten had made a complete recovery after 40 years. They had all had features typical of myalgic encephalomyelitis when they were ill. One had fallen ill in 1955, the others in 1948. Records indicated that the disease became endemic after the 1948 outbreak, so sporadic cases would have continued for years.

Eight out of the ten had a positive enterovirus VPI test; the two who were negative were the two who had made a complete recovery. Those people who had not made a complete recovery all had some degree of chronic handicap, although they themselves thought that they had made a good recovery. On psychological assessment, none of the ten showed any signs of neurosis or hysteria, they had all achieved satisfying lives or careers in spite of different amounts of disability.

Surely here is evidence to squash any remaining claims that ME is a psychological illness! In Iceland, Dr Hyde found people who had fallen ill forty years ago, who all conformed to the features of ME syndrome, and eight out of ten still have persisting enteroviral infection with persisting disabilities, and have overcome the handicaps of chronic illness quite successfully.

Summing up

So, after all these studies and theories, what is causing the ME syndrome?

(a) There is a persistent virus infection in most cases.
(b) Something has upset the immune response, possibly:

- a long past virus?
- a new virus?
- environmental factor, e.g. pesticides, chemical?
- stress?

(c) Maybe an inherited predisposition (ME diathesis).
(d) Physical exhaustion at the time of an infection seems to have an adverse effect (just as in polio).

Dr P. O. Behan suggested that ME is 'a metabolic disorder, caused by persistent virus infection and associated with defective immunoregulation'.

He wrote that in 1984. It is now 1988 and I do not think that a better description of the basic mechanism has been achieved. A lot of attention has been given to the virus aspect, and now future research needs to investigate what is causing the immune system disorder.

If, after reading this section about causes of ME, you are confused, it is because the picture of ME *is still* rather confused. There is no one single expert who can confidently explain exactly what causes ME, or exactly what is happening in our bodies. However, more and more pieces of the jigsaw are turning up each year; hopefully we shall soon see a complete picture, and then possibly a complete cure.

There may be some alarm and confusion arising from the publicity about AIDS and its causes, and a possible link with ME. In AIDS there is a total collapse of the patient's immune system, because the AIDS virus wipes out the lymphocytes, and there is no defence against infection. In ME the immune system is not working quite as it should, but there are plenty of lymphocytes, and the disease is quite different. If it was not, then ME patients would not still be around to suffer from their symptoms for five, ten, or 20 years!

Case History

The following history is an example of how the illness can keep reappearing over many years, the initial episode probably being a viral infection. It also illustrates the great variability of symptoms and hence the difficulty in diagnosis.

MR N. H. AGE 56 ARCHITECT

Mr H. was in Durban, South Africa in January and February of 1955. He picked up something that was going around, that was like severe flu, and was very ill. After a couple of months or so he recovered enough to return for his final year at the University of Cape Town. He did not know at the time about the outbreak of epidemic myalgic encephalomyelitis among the staff of Durban's Addington Hospital.

In 1961, while working in Aden, he developed an acute mental illness diagnosed as 'anxiety state', for which he was returned to the UK for treatment. The features of this mental illness resembled the anxiety and panic state suffered by many ME patients.

Then in 1978, in Cyprus,

> an older friend and I started to feel wobbly on our legs after a party at which we'd had only two drinks each. The feeling passed, then he but not I had a

very severe attack of a mysterious flu. He recovered, but after a while each of us began to get attacks of shakes, loss of balance, a tendency to throw a leg while walking, plus general lethargy, physical and mental. We went to various doctors with various diagnoses, which included atherosclerosis, brucellosis, and other things.

I returned to England, and the worst symptoms disappeared, but I had the lethargy and lack of concentration still and could not do my work properly. I went back to Cyprus in 1984 for one year, and found that my friend who had been ill at the same time six years earlier had deteriorated physically and mentally, and he subsequently died from some heart condition. I felt much worse in Cyprus, and the symptoms of loss of balance and shaking, plus fatigue, came back again.

Mr H. is settled in England since 1985. He continues to have mental and physical lethargy, aching, and pins and needles in the left hand. Other symptoms are: poor memory, varying eyesight, pain in the right thigh, great variability of all symptoms with ups and downs. He is unable to pursue his profession as an architect full-time, due to poor concentration and abnormal physical fatigability.

He has had extensive investigations carried out, in 1979, 1980, and 1983, with nothing abnormal found. In 1987 he was assessed by a new doctor, and other conditions being excluded was diagnosed as having ME.

He describes his condition with this analogy:

Myself with ME, and trying to do some work, is like a man and his car, where the man is the essential being with feelings, aspirations and so on; the car's engine is the physical brain that calculates, reasons, remembers and concentrates; and all the other parts of the car represent the body.

The car appears to be in good condition, always passes its MOT, and the engine starts first kick. Drive off and all goes well for a few miles, then the engine gets sluggish, the steering judders, the bodywork rattles and you have to pull into a lay-by. The man had been a taxi driver and sometimes is asked to drive somebody some distance.

Briefly forgetting the present he accepts because he always did and was glad to, but now he has the embarrassment of having to make the journey in short hops, inventing spurious reasons for stopping along the way.

Many mechanics had looked at the car but none had found anything wrong, until at last one new mechanic told the man that that particular model *did* suffer those defects and that they could not yet be put right. So it's a case of settling for doing local deliveries only.

Comment – Does Mr H.'s illness date from 1978, or from 1955? There was an epidemic of ME in Durban in 1955, though the cause of it was not isolated.

This man is not as seriously ill as many ME patients, but the easy fatigability and poor concentration has effectively terminated his professional career, and seems to originate either from a flu-like illness in 1978, or perhaps from a reactivation of something caught in Durban in 1955.]

4

ME – the Diagnosis

At the time of writing this book, there is no definitive test for ME which gives a clear **yes** or **no** in 100 per cent of suspected cases.

It has been suggested that, as there is no treatment, and you just have to live with it, there is no point in going to your doctor if you suspect you may have ME.

A recent TV programme in the UK set out to show that getting a diagnosis of ME had not helped those patients who had been selected to take part in the discussion. The arguments were not convincing; however the programme probably sowed seeds of doubt in the minds of many ME sufferers, who were on the brink of having their illness accepted by their GPs and families.

The point of diagnosis was brought home to me very forcibly, when, on the same day that this particularly unhelpful TV documentary was shown, I read a report of a young man who had just committed suicide. He had been ill for over a year with a 'chronic virus', had typical encephalitic symptoms of ME, and muscle fatigue. His work performance had deteriorated so much that his employers gave him notice to quit. The loss of job to someone who is struggling and ill, and is not recognized as such by employers – who should otherwise have discussed sick leave – can be the last and fatal straw.

So there are good reasons for you to seek a diagnosis if you think you may have ME:

(1) You need to rule out other conditions, some of which may be treatable – you may *not* have ME.
(2) You need the diagnosis, in order to apply for time off work or a change to part-time work, to apply for social security benefits, mobility allowance, home help, retirement pension, etc.
(3) If you are at school, you need the diagnosis to allow you to rest at home when ill, without your parents being prosecuted for your non-attendance. Yes, this does happen to parents of children with ME, though hopefully less now that the illness is better recognized.
(4) You need to know if you have a genuine illness in order to stay sane. To be told that your inability to stand up, to work normally, to think or live a normal life is *not* psychological is a wonderful relief, and may save some from suicide.
(5) Through knowing what is wrong, you can start to reorganize your life and come to terms with the illness.
(6) Getting a diagnosis is the starting point of improving for many. Battling on in ignorance of the problem is a sure way to get worse.
(7) You need all the support and understanding you can get. It is hard for your doctor, family and friends to supply this when they do not realize that you are really ill.
(8) The more experience your doctor has of patients with ME, the better his or her ability will be to help you and other sufferers.
(9) Through getting a diagnosis, you can be put in touch with others by means of patient organizations such as the ME Association.
(10) If you have *not* got ME, you may be very glad to

know it. Other possible reasons for tiredness, etc., can be explored and dealt with.

With so much publicity about the illness in the past year, a good number of people are going to their GPs to say, 'Have I got ME?' – people who may just be overtired or run down through inappropriate life style. This puts doctors in a quandary, because ME is not a disease which is taught in medical schools, or seen much in general hospital wards; there, if it is found, it is called something else, such as heart attack, abdominal pain, or nervous collapse of unknown cause.

The diagnosis is made on the history, and lack of objective signs of other disease. There are sometimes abnormal signs on physical examination of the nervous system, and there are a number of laboratory tests which may help confirm the diagnosis, but which, if normal, do not rule out ME.

A list of symptoms typical of ME is given in Chapter 1 (see pages 14–15). The cardinal symptom is **fatigue**, unrelieved by a short rest, made worse by exercise.

The following questionnaire was devised by Dr J. Richardson, a GP in the north-east of England. Dr Richardson has studied the illness in the many patients he has seen for over 30 years. As a self-assessment test, it gives an estimate of the likelihood of having ME, but does not replace a medical diagnosis.

Myalgic–Encephalitic Scoring Chart

		Score for answer Yes
1	Has there ever been any evidence, either illness or antibody level, of past viral infection?	1

2 Fatigue (evidence of myalgic involvement):

a) Are you less than 33 per cent efficient per day? This relates to a full day with hobbies after work, etc. — 2

b) Do you need a period of bed or settee rest during each day? or — 3

c) Do you need a period of bed or settee rest on two or three days each week? — 2

d) Have you excessive fatigue after work effort? — 2

3 Do you have nocturnal sweats or cold feelings? — 2

4 Do you have bizarre dreams? — 1

5 Evidence of disturbed mental activity:

a) Do you have difficulty in finding the correct words? — 1

b) Does your handwriting deteriorate if you write a long letter? — 1

c) Do you tire if you have to talk for long? — 1

6 Faint attacks:

a) Do you tend to have faint attacks and lose consciousness? — 3

b) Do you have attacks without loss of consciousness but have to sit or lie down? — 2

7	Do you have early morning fatigue?	1
8	Does noise, e.g. 'chatter', upset you?	1
9	Do you have cold or numb feelings in your extremities or face?	2
10	Is your gait consistent with your age or is it that of a much older or unsteady person?	1
	Maximum total	26

Note: 15 is the lowest score found, maybe perhaps 13.

If you go to your doctor, or to a specialist, do prepare some sort of history of your illness in writing, in advance. Write down:

- when you last felt well;
- all infectious illnesses you have had, especially any that occurred around the time of onset of symptoms;
- anything else that happened to you before the onset;
- if anyone in your family or work circle was ill at the same time, and if any of them developed symptoms of ME;
- your main symptoms that bother you now;
- if the symptoms have been steady, or if you have had spells without them;
- how your illness has affected your lifestyle, work, family life, etc.;
- how much exercise you could take when you were well, and what you can do now without ill effects;
- anything that seems to make you better.

This preparation will help the doctor, and save you from forgetting important information at the time of consultation – most ME sufferers have a bad memory which is worse when under cross-examination!

If possible, take with you a relative or close friend who knows you very well and who can add his or her observations about any changes in you, should your mind become a blank.

If your illness has begun shortly after a viral infection (sometimes up to six weeks later), and you have classical symptoms, then the diagnosis is fairly easy. It is much more difficult in someone who has become unwell gradually, with no obvious precipitating infection. For those people, it is especially helpful to try and remember past infections or bouts of unwellness, which may be as trivial-seeming as a 24-hour tummy bug while abroad.

Your doctor should inquire about childhood illnesses, previous health, operations, drugs taken, especially antibiotics, also about the health of your parents and siblings, and about family history of allergies, undue infections, or ME-type illness.

A full physical examination should be carried out, including blood pressure, examination of heart, lungs and abdomen, a search for enlarged glands, and tests of neurological function and muscle weakness.

There is rarely extreme muscle wasting, but there may be some loss of muscle bulk especially of the thighs. This is usually symmetrical, unless one limb is worse affected.

Neurological tests may show brisk tendon reflexes, but the plantar response is usually normal (the big toe curls down when the sole of the foot is lightly scratched) and there is no clonus (jerky contraction of a muscle when suddenly stretched). Two tests which are commonly abnormal are the vibration sense, and the Romberg test (sense of balance with eyes closed).

Simple tests of muscle power may be normal. However if muscles are exercised – such as the patient squeezing a rubber ball for one minute, or being sent to climb 40 stairs (if able!) – the muscles used will be found to be weak, the weakness lasting several hours or up to three days.

There is almost invariably muscle tenderness. Careful fingertip feeling of the thigh or upper back muscles usually reveals points of great tenderness.

A key factor in arriving at a diagnosis of ME is the exclusion of other diseases which might be causing fatigue. Briefly, these would include chronic infections, endocrine diseases, nervous system disorders, cancer, muscle diseases and the 'auto immune' disorders.

There are a number of blood tests which should be carried out, as well as urine testing and then possibly more specialized investigations for ME or to exclude other conditions. Muscle biopsies, electromyograms, and the enterovirus test are not routine tests at present. The enterovirus test may confirm the diagnosis, but there is a waiting-list of those wanting the test; it is only available at St Mary's Hospital, London at present, and even if it is negative, ME is not ruled out.

The diagnosis still rests on a careful history, and exclusion of other conditions. Once a doctor has seen a patient with ME, the symptom picture is not forgotten. It is fair to say that many doctors are unsure about recognizing the illness, or even believing in it, until they know one of their patients, one of the family or a colleague who develops it; this experience usually dispels any scepticism, and any other patients in the practice who have ME will benefit thereafter.

Details of the differential diagnosis, and a routine of investigations, one which is carried out by a consultant physician who is interested in ME, are given in Appendix B, which may be of interest to doctors and health workers.

Case Histories

The following stories show how lack of proper diagnosis adds to a patient's suffering.

MRS B. C. 34 YEARS OCCUPATION – CLERICAL

Ill for four years now. She has never been given any diagnosis other than 'anxiety and depression'.

Her illness came on suddenly, with severe sore throat. Some other people at work were also ill. She had several courses of *antibiotics*, none of which touched the throat infection, and she came out in red swollen rash all over. [Comment – a rash following antibiotics can occur in glandular fever.] She saw several doctors, none of whom diagnosed glandular fever, or anything else. Extensive blood tests and ECG tests were negative.

She had suffered from a 'mental breakdown' several years previously, and perhaps because of this, her GP put all her symptoms down to psychological causes. [Sadly, a common attitude of many doctors.]

> I have never really recovered from this infection, and have seen various specialists plus a psychiatrist, and more recently a hypnotherapist. I am told it is all 'anxiety and depression'. I find it hard to accept this diagnosis with such vivid symptoms, which are:

Chronic fatigue, heaviness in arms and legs, pains in joints, tingling in hands, irritability, mood swings, sluggish speech, find it difficult to write, nausea, bloating, indigestion, PMT, palpitations, itching, total disinterest in sex, fears and anxieties, insomnia, bad dreams, aching pain in face, strange taste in mouth, stinging eyes.

I saw a programme about ME, and recognized my illness. I have a past history of several severe attacks of urticaria; no one found out what I was allergic to.

If I went to my GP and suggested I had ME he would look at me in despair and think it was something else I had latched on to.

I feel strongly that my symptoms, which followed a severe virus infection, are *totally different* than before, when I had the depression.

I have not yet met anyone who understands when I try to describe the dreadful ghastly tired feeling which totally debilitates me. It is not even constant within a day. The very thought of doing anything exhausts me, yet I keep plodding on – it would be too easy to give in and do nothing. I feel a real achievement just to get through a day.

If I was *diagnosed* as ME I would have peace of mind, to know my symptoms were those of an illness and not of my imagination. It would help to know that others feel the same as I do.

[Comment – she *needs* to give in and do nothing. Not having any diagnosis, she is continuing to fight her fatigue and illness, therefore cannot even begin to get better.]

MRS C. M. AGE AT ONSET 63

One day in April 1982 I was ill passing water frequently, thought I had flu. Six days later I fainted several times and was taken to hospital – I wondered if it was a reaction to penicillin my GP had prescribed a few days earlier.

I had a high temperature, was very sick, fainted many times, felt light-headed and 'floating'. I had further sickness and diarrhoea, the temperature stayed high for over two weeks. Lots of blood tests, ECG, EEG, X-rays of kidney were done. The hospital discharged me, saying I'd had a virus.

I was very weak when I got home, could hardly walk, and had tingling down my arms, diarrhoea, nausea and dizziness. My GP thought the virus was affecting the inner ear, and gave Stemetil.

My health took a long time to improve, but I was very tired, no stamina, and spent much of the day in bed. Before my illness I was very active socially – now I had to give everything up, and felt much older. Some days I felt reasonably well, then suddenly would get weak muscles and tingling. I tried terribly hard to help myself – I stopped tea and coffee, took vitamins, glucose, yeast. I started skipping to try to strengthen the legs, and walking to the shops – I'd get there, but found it very difficult to get back. No one knows the effort I had to make sometimes to do quite simple things – such as having a bath or dressing.

Ten months after the original infection I collapsed, and in hospital they said I had cytomegalovirus and herpes in my blood, but these were not serious and shouldn't make me feel as ill as I did.

This muscle weakness and tiredness continued on and off. Sometimes I had diarrhoea, or dizziness, tingling arms and weak shaky legs.

I have never been given any diagnosis, only 'nerves'. Any attempt at mental activity leads to a feeling of confusion, I cannot carry heavy bags, some days I can hardly walk any distance. I am helped if I rest in bed for a few days.

I get depressed sometimes, but had some devastating family tragedies a few years ago. However I am convinced that the virus, or something, continued to affect me for years after the illness in April 1982, and still does.

5

Plan of Management

As you probably know, you cannot go to your doctor and come away with a prescription for a drug which will cure ME. Take comfort from knowing that most ME sufferers get better in time. There is good evidence to show that those who rest early in the illness have a better chance of recovery.

Present estimates are that if you have a diagnosis of ME and you have been ill for less than a year, you will have about a 70 per cent chance of recovery within five years. Of course this means that 30 per cent will still have ME after five years. However, this is an illness which usually has ups and downs, and if you can learn to manage your life with ME then you are unlikely to stay at the worst all the time. It is natural to remember only the worst times, the days when you feel absolutely awful, very depressed, and convinced that no one understands how ill you feel. But think also of the days when there has been a kind of lightness, an improvement in energy, the ability to breathe calmly and to think that life may still be good.

There are broadly three categories to describe the course of the illness:

(1) Patients who gradually get better, then stay better.
(2) Patients who have remissions and relapses (the remissions may last for several years), but never seem to shake the disease off permanently.

(3) A small number of unfortunate people in whom there is no remission, and who remain ill for years.

I have found it helpful, when going through a bad time, to refer back to a good day and to imagine myself in that happier state again. For this reason I think that keeping some sort of a **diary** is useful. Much has been said about the value of writing down all the bad symptoms as they occur, what you have eaten and drunk, and your activities – especially looking at exercise. In this way you may see a pattern develop, showing what things cause a relapse in you.

But it is just as important to commit to the diary the good days, the experiences which have given you pleasure or made you laugh, and any improvement in symptoms.

The diary can be kept in a cheap exercise book just as well as in a manufactured diary. As most ME sufferers have poor memories, a diary can be useful to refer to before going to see your doctor, and to look at the results of any therapies you have tried. It is best to try to develop a routine of scribbling something every morning or evening.

Even a weekly diary is useful. However, there are some people to whom the idea of monitoring their illness suggests that they might be hypochondriacs. This is understandable. The British in particular do not think it is quite 'the done thing' to take too much interest in one's aches and pains. However, if you take an interest in the good times as well as the bad times, then a bit of optimism may overcome the hypochondriasis.

Another good reason for keeping a record over a period of months is that it is hard to remember exactly how you were six months ago, and while there may be ups and downs the general trend is more likely to be one of very gradual improvement, which will only become obvious when you refer back to the diary.

Having said all this about a diary, I would like to reassure those ME people who cannot or simply don't wish to keep a record of an illness they would rather forget, that it is not an essential therapy; the ups and downs will still happen, though you may not see so clearly why they do. The decision to keep a diary is an individual one. If you are too ill to write, perhaps your carer can keep some sort of a record for you.

What has happened in a person with ME is a lessening of the body's defence system which deals with viral infection. Our state of being alive at all depends on continual adaptation of the body to outside influences – maintaining the body temperature, keeping the levels of nutrients and minerals (e.g. blood glucose and salt levels) in our tissues constant, supplying oxygen to all cells of the body, killing invading germs, repairing damaged tissue, etc. For a detailed account of how all this is achieved, you would need to study a book about physiology.

Factors Known to Decrease the Immune System Function

- *Virus infections* can cause a reduction in numbers and function of lymphocytes.
- *Ionizing radiation* – X-rays, nuclear fall-out.
- *Nutritional deficiencies* – especially lack of zinc, iron, essential fatty acids, protein, vitamins A, B_6, B_5 (pantothenic acid), C, E, and folic acid.
- *Smoking* depletes the body of vitamin C.
- *Refined carbohydrates*, i.e. glucose, sucrose and fruc-

tose, reduce available vitamin C and impair white cell function.
- *Certain drugs* such as steroids, anti-cancer drugs, the contraceptive pill, possibly some antibiotics (by upsetting the natural balance of friendly bacteria in the body) and immuno-suppressants used after transplants.
- *Stress* – especially if protracted. This includes physical stress such as exposure to cold or exhaustion, and mental or emotional stress such as bereavement, over-worry, divorce.

Recent research has shown a definite link between psychological stress and immune functioning (*Lancet*, June 1987). What seems to be relevant is not the amount of stress one is exposed to, but how one handles it; thus someone who remains depressed for a long time after a bereavement or serious family illness has a greater chance of becoming ill themselves. So the observation by many ME sufferers that they thought they had undue stress for a period before developing ME is logical. If severe stress had led to their immune system not working so efficiently, then their bodies would not be able to deal with a viral infection properly.

The aim of any plan of management of ME should be to encourage the body to mobilize its own healing forces. We have an amazing capacity for healing and repair of damage in our bodies; unfortunately, for all sorts of reasons, this healing force is often suppressed, as explained above. Anything that will allow the immune system to become stronger and to overcome the persistence of viruses in our cells, should be valuable for an ME sufferer.

A person with ME has little energy. Therefore it is vital that none is wasted on unnecessary activity. This includes physical activity, worry and anxiety, and the energy required for digesting the wrong foods, and for dealing with chemicals in food, drink, or the air we breathe.

If the immune system is having to deal with other foreign agents, it will not have enough resources to deal effectively with a continuing viral infection. And if the ME sufferer also has allergic reactions to foods and chemicals, the stresses caused by these allergies further reduce the energy available for healing.

It may help to visualize your state of health as resulting from the balance between things that decrease your healing energy, and those things that promote recovery.

Negative Factors	*Positive Factors*
Too much exercise	Physical rest
Lack of sleep	Sleep
Worry	Freedom from anxiety
Mental strain	Mental rest
Work stress	Relaxation
Sadness, bereavement	Calmness
Loneliness	Love and friendship
Cold and damp	Warmth
Hunger	Joy, laughter
Wrong food	Good nourishing food
Sudden shocks	Fresh air and sunshine
Surgery	Lack of chemical pollution
Most drugs	Avoiding infection
Anaesthetics	Patience and optimism
Infections	
Poisons (alcohol, chemicals, smoking, pollution, etc.)	

If you look at these lists, you can see that all the positive factors are the sort of things we try to give our children and those we love. When you are ill, you need to spoil yourself a bit, to give yourself those good and natural things you would wish for a loved one. It is not realistic to expect others to provide them all, though if you have love and support from others it is a tremendous help; but you *can* organize quite a lot of positive forces for yourself.

In planning a campaign for learning to live with ME it is best to do it in stages, and have an order of priority. There is not yet enough evidence that the following suggestions will be helpful in every case, however stopping exercise and resting seem to be essential for all sufferers. Other lines of management have *all helped some people*.

The advice offered in this book is not aimed at achieving a cure of ME, but rather to lessen the severity, encourage more remissions, and help you to live more comfortably with the condition.

It is not much use spending money and time on various treatments and at the same time continuing to live a busy lifestyle – so **rest** is the very first thing to organize!

Things to do to help you cope with ME

- Organize your lifestyle to allow you more rest
- Stop all unnecessary exercise
- Learn to relax – e.g. meditation
- Accept your limitations
- Improve your nutrition
- Keep warm
- Take nutritional supplements especially vitamin C
- Avoid chemical pollution

- Deal with candida infection if present
- Treat any allergies
- Have more fresh air and daylight
- Avoid low blood sugar
- Learn to handle depression
- Develop positive thinking and serenity (of course this is difficult on bad days!)
- Do not be shy to ask for help
- Apply for things to make life easier (social services help, walking-aids, etc.)
- Consider other therapies such as massage or homeopathy
- Contact other sufferers for support if you feel isolated
- Consider joining a local ME group
- Do not compare yourself with other ME people, some will be more ill, some less.

In learning to live with ME, half the battle is won if you can *accept* that you just *cannot* live at the same pace as you did before you became ill. To do this you need to realize that your worth is not measured by achievements in terms of being busy, earning money, athleticism or even being good at anything!

'He also serves who only stands and waits' is a good motto to remember – but substitute 'sits' or 'lies' for 'stands'.

Remember you will probably improve.

Also remember that of all the suggestions listed here, **physical and mental rest** and **good nutrition** are the most important. The following chapters will talk about these things in more detail.

6
The Importance of Rest and Sleep

A person with ME is like a battery that cannot hold its charge. The battery can be connected to charging leads overnight, and in the morning it appears to be full of energy, but after very little use the lights go dim, the engine won't turn over, and the only solution is to recharge it. Of course you can buy a more efficient battery, but you have to make do with the human body. So rest is all about recharging batteries.

The metabolic machinery in an ME sufferer has gone wrong. Energy is taken into the body via food, and oxygen in the inspired air, but the transformation of it into useful energy output seems to be quite inefficient. For reasons which are not yet scientifically clear, there is a 'spanner in the works' of the power house in each body cell which is affected by the ME illness, and the cells which most obviously show up this defect are those of muscle and brain.

In the power house of a cell affected by ME the amount of RNA is reduced, and the rate of replenishment of it is also reduced (see page 45). As RNA is part of the mechanism that develops power, the function of that cell will be inefficient, and it takes longer to recover. This applies to brain cells as well as muscle cells. When you use muscles, a by-product of the energy reaction is lactic acid, and a build up of lactic acid in the muscle causes pain. In a healthy muscle you only get lactic acid build up if you over-use a muscle that is not developed for that use, e.g. a game of tennis when you are unfit. This pain and stiffness normally disappears in a day or two in a healthy person. But the ME affected muscle accumulates lactic acid after relatively little work, and also takes far longer to get rid of it and recover. Even walking around the house or getting out of bed may be enough to maintain the lactic acid and pain and tenderness in the legs virtually continuously.

If you start to feel exhausted, mentally or physically, there is absolutely no point in pushing yourself on, as the stage of complete collapse will soon arrive. Many sufferers find out by experience that more can be achieved in a day by doing only a little at a time, and having frequent rests, than by pushing on to the limit and then having to have a long rest. The great problem in managing exercise and rest is that by the time you feel exhausted, you may have passed the stage at which a short rest might have recharged you. By the time you feel completely 'done in', it may take several days of rest to recover. If you stop before this point, recovery may only take a few hours.

Therefore a daily routine, in which you can do things in a rhythm of activity and rest, worked out to suit **you**, is recommended. During a period of severe illness or relapse, the daily activity may be merely several trips to the bathroom and perhaps a short time in a chair by a window. Someone in a better state may be able to work for a few hours, then rest, then eat lunch, rest again, work a bit more, rest, cook supper, etc.

However unwell you may be, you are likely to have a daily pattern to your energy – some wake up feeling reasonably human, but steadily run down as the day progresses; these people need to plan to do things such as phone calls, socializing, cooking, letter writing, etc., early in the day, to make most efficient use of what energy there is. Many others wake up (if they have slept) feeling they would rather be dead, and by later on they may improve. For them, things to be done should be arranged for a later time of day. It is worth telling friends and colleagues when to call, and when not to bother you. This saves you the awkwardness of being incoherent on the phone to someone you would otherwise love to talk to.

If you are well enough to think of working part-time, and this can be arranged, it obviously pays to try and organize your working hours to suit your best time of day. This will be less stressful on both you and your colleagues, as well as more efficient. Having said all this, I do realize that there are sufferers who find no pattern to their levels of energy at all. However, if you keep a diary of ups and downs and of what you have been doing, then some sort of pattern may well emerge.

Rest

The more you rest early on in the illness or during a relapse, the quicker you will improve.

Resting, and the giving up of a lot of activities which were part of a busy life, requires discipline. In this decade of the twentieth century, we have been bombarded with exhortations to take exercise in order to be healthy. The streets and parks are full of joggers, friends always seem to be planning 'activity' holidays such as ski-ing, sailing, or walking. We are conditioned now to think that if you sit all day in a chair you will become ill or get furred up arteries, and for a healthy person this may be true. Success tends to be measured by visible achievement; 'keeping busy' is reckoned to be good for one's morale; people who live 18-hour days and give the impression of being healthy and successful are much admired.

If you have ME you must unlearn all these conditionings. You will have to learn to be a Mary instead of a Martha, an observer and listener instead of a doer or talker!

In spite of all that I have learned about viruses, immune systems, or chemical reactions in the body, I have a sneaking feeling that I regard ME as something which has come along to force me to step out of the busy world for a time, a sort of desperate plea from my body to get me to put the brakes on and just stop. This mechanism of course does not apply to all sufferers, some of whom may consider that their lives were calm and unhurried anyway before they got ME, so that there was no need for it to happen to them.

Do try and think of the giving up of activities as something **positive**, to do, rather than **negative** and giving in to ME. Rest should be regarded as positive, constructive treatment rather than just as 'doing nothing'. In restructuring your life, you will find that you have a spring-clean of priorities, and in fact some aspects of life become much simpler, because there will be fewer choices to have to make.

For example: if you do not have the energy (or money) to go shopping for clothes, you will not have those exhausting hours trying to decide what garment best suits you, and as you do not go out so much, the clothes you have will be quite adequate. If you cannot cook large meals or entertain, you do not have to worry about those people you think you ought to invite – your good friends will come and visit you, and the others can wait until you are better.

Contentment and happiness can come from very

simple things. With a debilitating illness, the secret of coping is to lower your sights, *to move the goalposts a lot nearer*. Then you will be able to score an achievement more often, with a great deal less effort. Then a walk to a local shop can be as exciting as a weekend walking in the country. An evening spent looking at a sunset can give as much pleasure as a trip to the cinema.

A friend visited me recently who had not seen me for two years. He said, 'Poor you, how the quality of your life has suffered because of this ME thing!' He remembered me as someone who had a fulfilling and busy job, walked everywhere, and enjoyed mountaineering. To my surprise I found myself contradicting him; I described how I had watched the development of spring in close detail, how many books I had been able to read, the time now available to write to overseas friends, the rich variety of programmes on the radio. This sounds rather smug, and of course I have had times when I have been angry about being unable to walk, and also very depressed about it all. I really believe that I did not begin to get better until I stopped being frustrated by the disability, stopped worrying about money, and started making the most of the new type of existence. I also realize that many people with ME are too ill even to be able to read, or to listen to the radio, and for them it is obviously hard to find much quality in life.

I can hear many of you say, having read these last paragraphs: 'It's all very well for you, but I've small children, how can I rest?'; 'They cannot do without me at work'; or 'We have a mortgage to pay, how can I go on sick leave?'

Well, you have a valid point. But have you really considered all the possible ways of asking for help? Most people like to give help and are waiting to be asked. There may be a forgotten relative who could help, or a lonely neighbour who would be very happy to do some shopping or look after the children sometimes. It is worth asking your doctor, or the citizens' advice bureau, what sorts of help are available, such as home help and various disability benefits. Do remember that your health is more precious than money, and that none of us are indispensable at work. The office, clients, patients, workshop, etc., will all be there when we get better. So will the possibility of doing many other things, even if you have to give up the job you had when you became ill.

Obviously each sufferer must decide how best to reorganize life. It is usually a question of sorting out the priorities, the most important of which has to be 'to get better'.

I have a scarlet sweat-shirt with a motif on it, 'Non Omnia Possumus Omnes' – which is Latin for 'It is not possible to do everything!' It was acquired before this present illness, but I find it a useful garment to wear when I'm tempted to overfill my day . . .

In the early stages of the illness, as much rest as possible should be obtained. At this time one should not try to do anything more than the bare minimum. Some people worry about loss of muscle bulk and power from lack of use. In fact the shrinking of muscles is not as great as one would expect, nothing like the wasting that happens in paralytic diseases such as polio. However, if you are ill enough to be spending all day in bed, and if this is likely to be for weeks, then it is sensible to do some very simple and non-strenuous movements each day. Every joint should be moved through its full range, to avoid the development of contractures or a stiff joint; and gentle stretching of the whole body should be attempted, as is done by a cat on waking. This can be done yourself or very gently by a carer.

Suggested movements

- *Shoulders*: lift each arm slowly forwards, up beside the ears, back as far as possible, and down.
- *Elbows*: straighten each arm completely, then bend so that the hand touches the shoulder.
- *Wrists*: keeping the forearm still, make a circle with the finger tips.
- *Fingers*: curl them up, then straighten them, spread them wide.
- *Neck*: starting with the chin on the chest, make a slow circle of the chin in both directions, so that the neck bends forwards, then sideways, then backwards, to the other side, then forward again.
- *Hips*: lying prone or on the side, take the leg backwards, return to starting place, then take it sideways. These movements need not be great, but are important to prevent the hips becoming stiff and bent.
- *Knees*: gently straighten the legs from time to time.
- *Ankles*: circle the foot in each direction.
- *Back*: Lying prone for a while each day should extend the back. Back tension can be eased a bit by bringing the knees to (or near) the chin, then unfolding again.

The object of these movements is *not* to strengthen muscles, but is to prevent stiffness or deformity of joints. Most patients will be doing enough each day for this immobility not to become a problem – e.g. having a bath, drying, putting on clothes, walking round the house. Even if you have to spend most of the day in or on the bed, it is suggested that you change out of the nightclothes into something else which is warm and comfortable during the day. This is psychologically good, and also moves the joints!

There is a narrow margin between lying in bed and doing absolutely nothing, and maintaining enough mobility to keep the body supple while still having enough rest. The other reason for moving around is to keep some circulation going to the extremities, which tend to get cold anyway.

Sleep

This is the best form of rest. During sleep the rate of repair of body tissue is greatest. Animals and children sleep the clock round when they are ill. Many ME patients complain that they seem to need too much sleep, but you should allow yourself to sleep as much as you can, it will do nothing but good. If you don't sleep well, you cannot get well.

Unfortunately a good night's sleep is hard to achieve for many sufferers. All sorts of things conspire to prevent it: muscle or joint pains, oversensitivity to noise, twitchings, palpitations, sweating, nightmares, breathing difficulties, panic attacks, and a racing brain that just will not switch off even though you feel exhausted.

So if you have chances to sleep in the day, take them. Use any means you find useful to get some sleep at night. If you expect to spend some time awake during the night, have some distraction at hand, such as a radio or silly book, and also something to eat, and try not to fret about being awake. Getting upset about insomnia wastes energy and stops one relaxing.

Suggestions for helping you to sleep

- Go to bed before you become exhausted and allow time to relax, e.g. with quiet radio or an easy book.

- Make sure your bed is comfortable. If the muscles are very sore, put a quilt, duvet or sleeping bag under the lower sheet. If you are spending most of the time in bed, consider investing in a washable sheepskin to lie on. The mattress should be fairly soft but not sagging. I have found a good quality latex foam (non-inflammable) mattress better than a sprung one, and also better insulated and hence warmer, but this is a personal preference.
- Make sure you are warm enough. Chilliness increases muscle tension. An electric blanket, switched off before you go to sleep, is a boon for aching limbs even in our so called 'summer'.
- Essential oils, especially lavender, in the bath or gently massaged into the limbs, really do help. If you can get someone else to do this for you, even better. You can find out more about the properties of various oils by consulting an aromatherapist or reading a book on the subject. It is important to use only oils that are calming or relaxing – those that are stimulating should be avoided. Lavender seems to be good for most ME people, it relaxes and calms muscles and balances body energies.
- Avoid exciting or distressing TV, radio programmes, or books in the evening. If one is emotionally fragile, one can weep through the night about some tragedy seen on the news.
- Do not go to sleep hungry, for you will wake up between 2 a.m. and 4 a.m. feeling awful – hence the snack ready in case.
- Make sure the bedroom is properly ventilated; there does not need to be a howling gale from the window, but an airtight stuffy room does not provide enough oxygen, and may increase indoor air pollution.
- Ear-plugs are a boon if you are extra noise sensi-

tive, and will muffle street noises, courting cats, ticking clocks and snoring spouses. The best are the soft wax ones, which soften in the ear, fit snugly, and are non-irritant. They are also useful on a noisy train or bus, or in any situation when noise is an irritation. In summer they can be at hand when resting in the garden, to put in if a neighbouring lawn mower starts up.

- Avoid having lots of electric flexes passing across or near the bed-head, and if possible switch things off at the plug before sleeping, except for a bedside light. Electromagnetic energy fields may not affect healthy people, but many ME sufferers seem to be extra sensitive to them, and sleep disturbance may be one of the effects.
- There are various herbal teas available which are mildly sedative and non-addictive, e.g. chamomile, and special night-time mixtures. Avoid tea or coffee after 4 p.m., if you still drink these. If milk does not disagree, then an old-fashioned warm milky drink at bedtime is worth trying. Heated milk contains calcium and tryptophan (an amino acid, a component of protein), which are both sedative, and the calories help prevent night starvation.
- Tryptophan can be taken as 500 mg tablets, one or two about an hour before bedtime. It should not be taken with milk or any other protein. It is non-addictive and sedative. It can also be helpful in some cases of depression, in which case the dose may be higher. (See Chapter 14, page 203.)
- *Sleeping pills* are probably best avoided, as they can lead to dependence on them, and they have to be broken down by the liver, which may not be working perfectly. However, if nothing else works, and you are suffering night after night, and

feeling exhausted in the morning, then taking a mild sedative for a few weeks may be the lesser of two evils. Once you start to feel a bit better you may be able to do without them. A short-acting one like Temazepam 5mg to 10mg should give six to seven hours of sleep and not make you groggy in the morning.

- Most anti-depressants are sedative, some more than others. They would not normally be prescribed for insomnia unless your doctor considers that your insomnia is due to depression. However for intractable sleep disturbance, a low dose of an anti-depressant such as doxepin (sinequan) 10–25mg at night can be useful. However some cannot tolerate the side effects of anti-depressants. (See Chapter 14.)

In the early stages of the illness or during a relapse, the symptoms that result from doing too much develop within a few hours or the next day. With recovery, the time lapse from overdoing it to getting the symptoms (that prove that you shouldn't have done it) gets longer and it becomes more difficult to relate cause and effect. The muscle pain, weakness, sweating or feeling awful may not happen until several days following the imprudent exertion. If you are still keeping a diary it may show you what has caused the relapse. With recovery, the length of time needed to come out of a relapse should get shorter, maybe one week of rest instead of three months; maybe one day instead of a week.

Beware – during the time of gradual recovery, it is very tempting, when feeling so wonderfully well (comparatively), to forget you still have ME and to do something stupid like running for a bus or shifting furniture. I know some people whose sudden extreme exertion has put them back to bed for *months*.

Getting better with ME is like a game of snakes and ladders, but at least you have some control over the fall of the dice.

There are various levels of rest, ranging from weeks in bed to an hour sitting in a chair. But it is very important to have mental and emotional rest as well as physical rest. Most of us have a constant chatter of thoughts whizzing around in the brain while we are awake.

If you are used to a busy job (and I include running a home), then quite likely when you were well you were able to have three levels of thought going on at once.

For example: the most conscious level is holding a conversation; the middle level is composing a shopping list; the deep level is worrying about some unsolvable problem such as your child's bad school progress. Familiar?

Now when you have ME this sort of mental acrobatics is nearly impossible and leads to confusion and brain fatigue. The short-term memory goes, so by the time you reach the third item on the shopping list you have forgotten the first two. You struggle wearily upstairs to get something, only to forget what it is you wanted. Simple decisions become difficult, probably because the circuits which would normally go click-click in the brain and arrive at an answer are not functioning.

It is no good trying to force your brain to cope. Many of the circuits and terminals in the computer in your head are out of order because of the virus. Some days more circuits will function than others. Computer experts have coined the term 'virus trouble' to describe some mysterious malfunctions in computer systems. I wonder if these boffins have experience of ME?

You should learn to concentrate on just one thing at a time. I find it helpful to have a notebook by me, one in every room, in which to jot down things that I have just thought of, and to put things in writing before they are quickly forgotten. Then of course you have to remember where you put the notebooks!

The frustration and rage at the lack of brain function is very wasteful of mental energy, and for previously mentally agile patients this can be harder to bear than the physical fatigue. If the confusion comes on quickly during the day, it may signal the need for some food and/or a rest. The best thing to do if a sudden fog comes over you is to stop whatever you are trying to do, have something to eat if it is three hours or more since the last meal, and have a little doze. Many ME people manage to stay in a job by negotiating a flexibility of hours and arranging a couch to rest on if their energy suddenly runs out.

The same principles of stopping before you reach complete exhaustion apply to brain fatigue as to muscle tiredness. For months I simply could not cook a simple meal at 6 p.m., and I struggled and swore in the kitchen, and cried over the difficulty of co-ordinating brain and hands and cooker even to boil potatoes. Then I started to have a snack at 4 p.m. followed by a pre-cooking rest, and now the evening meal is generally edible and I am not too weary to eat it.

There is a way to help the mind rest, it is called meditation, a way of resting body and mind that has been practised for centuries. Meditation is recommended for ME patients and is discussed in detail in Chapter 12.

How does one achieve emotional rest? This is difficult because ME causes emotional fragility anyway. When people or events make you upset, try and learn to say to yourself, 'It doesn't matter, it can't hurt me.'

Living with ME can strengthen our inner resources, lead us to be less dependent on the opinions and approval of others. If one can imagine a protective coat around one's heart, then perhaps 'the slings and arrows' of life might have less power to hurt. However, the worst sling or arrow for many of us is having ME.

A friend with ME told me, 'I try not to react to upsetting things now, nor to get overexcited or over-happy. I have reduced the level of all emotional reactions and just let things wash past me, and it is easier to cope.'

It is easy and common for friends and family of sufferers to cause hurt. One finds out who the real friends are, many others melt away because they feel threatened by the illness – people ask, 'Can I catch it from you?', and are not convinced when I say, 'No.' They do not know how to approach someone who has changed and whose mood may be unpredictable. The upset from such hurt can be lessened if one has a strong belief in oneself, and if one can realize that one's soul, personality, or whatever you call it, is still intact and special, in spite of ME and losing friends.

Do remember that when you have ME, all your functions need to be adjusted so as not to waste precious energy, i.e. physical activity, mental work, and emotional reactions. You need to work out new patterns of behaviour, and to do this effectively you need to listen to what your body and mind are telling you.

'One way of looking at the illness is to see it as our body going on strike, and demanding new terms and conditions of employment. Most people with ME are by nature highly energetic and people tend to look to them for support and enthusiasm. ME seems to thrive on these patterns of behaviour' (from an article by a patient). It may be that a lot of ME people will not make any real progress until certain patterns of living have been unlearned, and other more energy-conserving behaviour has been learned.

Getting ME is a clear message that something is wrong. The virus has forced you to come to a full stop, and fighting what is happening is the worst thing you can do. So give in gracefully, stop fighting yourself, rest, rest, and rest some more and let the world go by for a time. Unless you do this, the disease is likely to take an even deeper hold.

Case History

The following story is told by a lady who has had ME for 18 years.

MISS W. T. AGE NOW 67 RETIRED

I was first ill in 1970, aged 49. It was thought at the time to be a virus infection, there were a number of funny viruses around at the time.

There were years of 'relapse and recovery', years of weak legs, years of apparent good health, and a steady decline starting winter of 1982–3, until summer 1985 (when I started to adapt my life instead of trying to fight it). Since then the only relapses have been when I was in hospital for tests and forced to exercise for physiotherapy or testing. For the last two years I have been able to live at barely 50% of normal life.

Symptoms – worst in relapse
Muscle weakness, causing problems with standing, walking, carrying. Fatigue. Pain and jumpy legs at night, sensitivity to noise, inability to concentrate

for long, sleep disturbance – brain may race and I cannot relax, or I may go to sleep, then wake feeling disturbed by a bad dream. Very sensitive to changes of temperature, words get muddled.

When I am very tired, I am very clumsy and irritable, and my face goes a nasty yellow-grey colour.

Medical tests done (many)
For glandular fever, normal; for underactive thyroid, normal.
Gland biopsy. Repeated tensilon tests – normal.
Muscle biopsy – showed slight abnormality.
Repeated electromyograms – normal, one slightly abnormal. Skull X-ray and CT scan – normal.
Psychological interview – normal!

Diagnoses
1970, 1972, 1976 – 'virus infections'
1984 – 'nothing wrong with you'
1985 – damage to nerve in muscle, ? cause (from muscle biopsy)
1986 – nothing neurologically wrong, advised to see a psychiatrist!
Later 1986 (same muscle biopsy) – damage to muscle, could be due to earlier virus?
1986 – ME (after 17 years!)

I worked out that the muscle weakness dated from the old virus infection (1970), but doctors would not listen to me. In 1986 I heard a radio talk about ME, it sounded like me. I sent off to the ME Association for more information, I became more convinced. Later I found a consultant who is familiar with ME, who confirmed the diagnosis, without doing further tests.

In the light of my experience during the last four years, I cannot stress too much the need for rest, and for adopting a lifestyle in keeping with one's limitations. Right from getting the initial virus, I wanted to keep going and was encouraged to be as active as possible as soon as possible. Since my troubles really started in about 1984, doctors have continually told me to keep going, and even when I was diagnosed as having irreparable damage and told by my GP to adapt my lifestyle and keep within my limits, the neurologist was still assuring me that I must *not* rest, I must keep as active as ever possible.

It was during the time that I was fighting against the weakness, and dragging myself about in an effort to keep going, that my condition deteriorated so fast and so permanently. As soon as I modified my life and listened to what my body was saying and kept within my limits whatever anyone said, it was amazing how the deterioration slowed down and almost stopped.

The ME Association theory is that rest in the initial stages can be a big factor in recovery. I never had that rest. And now, I cannot help wondering whether, if I had been advised to rest even in 1984, instead of being instructed to keep going, I might not have the permanent damage which has now occurred.

7

Good Nutrition for ME

Why is good nutrition so important for someone with ME?

(1) Because there may be deficiencies of essential nutrients present for a long time, due to poor diet or stress earlier in life.
(2) Because digestion and absorption of food may be impaired. This may be caused by lack of digestive enzymes resulting from viral damage to the pancreas, candida infection, or damage to the cell lining of the small intestine.
(3) Because liver function may be impaired, and the liver has to deal with any non-nutrients in the diet.
(4) Because protein, essential fats, and certain minerals and vitamins need to be well supplied, for the immune system to work properly.

Changing and improving the diet is, for many sufferers, one of the simplest ways of affecting progress with ME. A special anti-candida diet is described in Chapter 9.

Guidelines for Basic Healthy Eating

- Eat regular meals, do not miss breakfast or lunch.
- Use unprocessed wholefoods – avoid dried, packaged, dehydrated, or canned food.

- Avoid all refined carbohydrates, i.e. sugar (brown or white), white flour, polished rice, white pasta.
- Avoid alcohol, coffee, tea (except weak tea in moderation), cola drinks, chocolate.
- Have good quality protein at least once, preferably twice a day.
- Have plenty of fresh fruit and vegetables.

Have vegetables raw in salads at least once a day, and if cooked, cook lightly in minimal water or steam, to avoid losing precious minerals – except for potatoes.

Peel or wash all fruit with skins, thoroughly wash all vegetables, unless you know they are grown without any chemicals or sprays. Try and use them as fresh as possible.

Be more adventurous with salads, using sprouted legumes (e.g. bean sprouts), grated carrot, grated beetroot, shredded cabbage, etc., in winter when the traditional salad stuff is out of season. If you already possess a food processor, you should make full use of it to prepare finely chopped salads and thick vegetable soups.

If you can afford it, you might consider investing in a *juicer*, which extracts much more of the enzymes, vitamins and minerals from living plants, than can be obtained by liquidizing or squeezing them. Very highly nutritious drinks of fruit and vegetable juice can be made, leaving only the undigestible cellulose behind. You would need to eat a very large volume of the plants to get the equivalent amount of juice.

Juiced fruits or vegetables are ideal for someone whose appetite is very poor, or for someone who is alone and too unwell to chop or peel things.

Vegetables and fruit are extremely important, not only to supply a good level of vitamin C daily, but to give many other essential nutrients, which are other vitamins, minerals and essential fats. There is great value in eating some food raw daily, as some enzymes and vitamins are destroyed in cooking.

Protein

Protein is made up of amino acids. These are the building blocks used for repair and replacement of body cells. They are also essential for making antibodies to infection, neuro-transmitters, hormones and the various lymphokines produced by the immune system. Some amino acids can be made in our bodies, others have to be supplied in food, and are therefore termed 'essential'.

There are eight essential amino acids. For any diet to be adequate in its protein supply, it must give enough of all the essential amino acids.

'First class' proteins contain all the essential amino acids in the right balance. These are proteins derived from animal sources: meats, fish, eggs, milk products.

'Second class' proteins are deficient in one or more of the essential amino acids, and come from plants. However, by combining plant proteins properly, all the amino acids are supplied, e.g. rice and lentils, wheat and beans.

Although meat is traditionally regarded as a good protein food, it does have two drawbacks.

(1) It is high in animal fat, i.e. saturated fat, the kind we are not supposed to have too much of.
(2) Unless you obtain meat from animals that have been 'organically' reared, or from free-range animals and wild game, you risk consuming hormones and antibiotics.

So the best meats are:

- free-range chicken, which is low in fat if you remove the skin, and turkey
- venison, rabbit, grouse, hare, partridge, etc. These roam free and are not kept confined, so have no additives, and are low in fat.
- lamb, especially mountain lamb (sheep are usually free-ranging), but it is not low in fat.
- organ meats from organically raised animals, liver, heart, kidneys, etc. These are low in fat and very rich in other nutrients as well as protein.

Fish is an excellent food, it is complete protein, it contains fish oils, which are a good source of unsaturated fats, and is also a good source of iodine and zinc. Even if you do not eat animal meat, it is a good idea to have fish at least twice a week.

Eggs are an excellent food because, even though an average egg contains only 7–8 gm of protein, it is a complete protein and easily digested. Eggs are also a good source of cholesterol, B vitamins, vitamins A and E, and zinc. Eggs from free-ranging chickens are superior in flavour, nutrient content, and freedom from additives.

Milk and milk products (if you are not allergic to them) are good – skimmed milk is better than full cream milk as the percentage of protein is higher and fat is less. The best cheeses are those with no added yellow colour, and low fat. Plain, live yoghourt is excellent as a source of protein and calcium, and has the organisms needed for proper balance in the colon.

Have protein daily, at two meals at least. In ME, it is essential to have a good intake of all essential amino acids for any recovery to take place. There is often poor digestion of proteins, because the pancreas is involved in the viral infection, with consequent deficiency of the pancreatic enzymes needed to break down protein into small enough peptides for absorption. Because of this, many sufferers have found it helpful to take supplements of amino acids, especially if they have frequent digestive and bowel problems. There are, however, a few whose digestion cannot handle protein from animal sources, and who therefore need to eat a lot of vegetable proteins. They may be better able to cope with protein by taking pancreatic enzymes. Meat is more digestible if it is cooked long and slowly (e.g. casseroled).

There is controversy over the suitability of a vegetarian diet for someone with ME. It depends a great deal on what you are used to, and how you feel on a high meat diet. It is possible to have enough high quality protein as a lactovegetarian (i.e. eating vegetables and dairy products), but it is nearly impossible to manage on a vegan diet if you have ME.

A vegan diet avoids all animal or dairy products, thus relying exclusively on protein from grains, pulses and nuts. This may be fine if you are well, but many ME sufferers are intolerant of wheat, and also have problems digesting pulses in any quantity, due to lack of digestive enzymes. So a vegan diet tends to cause extra bloating, abdominal pain and gas, as well as risking deficiencies of essential amino acids, vitamin B_{12}, vitamin D, zinc, iron, and calcium. Soya products – soya milk, tofu – are used in a vegan diet and contain calcium and protein, however it is easy to develop an intolerance or allergy to soya, if there is any allergic tendency.

So for all these reasons, *a vegan diet is not recommended* to anyone trying to get better from ME.

It is not a good idea, when you are ill, to become a vegetarian if you are accustomed to fish and meat, nor suddenly to eat a lot of fish and meat if you have been a vegetarian for some time. Sudden changes like these mean that the digestive system and liver have to adapt, and they may not do so very well.

Carbohydrates

These provide the main fuel for energy supply. Someone doing hard exercise daily, such as a labourer or athlete, needs plenty of carbohydrate to burn for energy. An ME sufferer will need much less.

Refined carbohydrates are pure starch or sugar, from which the husk and germ have been largely removed by refining. They are quickly digested and absorbed, and tend to lead to a rapid rise in blood glucose level, which is usually followed in two or three hours by a rapid drop in blood glucose, due to the release of insulin from the pancreas in response to the glucose rise. (See Chapter 13.)

It is much better for the blood glucose level *not* to go up and down in surges, as this puts stress on the pancreas, liver, and adrenals, and leads to unpleasant symptoms of faintness, sick hunger and irritability.

Refined carbohydrates provide 'empty calories', i.e. calories but no other nutrients. The valuable nutrients, protein, fat, B vitamins and minerals have been removed.

Complex carbohydrates are the starch together with the husk and seed-germ, such as wholewheat, unrefined oats, brown rice, potatoes with their skins, wholewheat pasta. They are more slowly digested, leading to a more gradual rise in blood glucose, and also provide essential fibre and nutrients. With complex carbohydrates you have to eat a lot more in volume to give the same amount of energy as refined carbohydrate. To get 250 cals of energy you can eat a small bar of chocolate, or four slices of wholemeal bread!

Sugar is called 'pure, white and deadly' with good reason. It is unnecessary, and a relatively recent addition to our diets in the evolution of man. The too high consumption of sugar in sweets, chocolates, cakes, breakfast cereals, tea and coffee, and in canned drinks (a can of coke contains seven teaspoons of sugar!) is responsible not only for dental decay, but for obesity, diabetes, heart disease and many other disorders which may include immune deficiency.

Honey is still a sugar, and only marginally better, as it contains minute amounts of minerals and vitamins. However it is mostly sucrose and fructose.

Fats

We are being urged to reduce our fat consumption as part of a healthier diet. What is more important is to change the ratio of kinds of fat, and to have more 'essential fats' and less saturated fats, which are mostly of animal source.

Essential fatty acids

These are found in good quality polyunsaturated oils and margarines, nuts and seeds, most vegetables, and in fish, especially oily fish.

They are essential for life. Apart from needing fat as a store of available energy and for insulation, we need essential fatty acids because they form the main structure of cell membranes and walls in every body cell; they are also needed to make highly active substances which are vital for all body functions. These include hormones (the sex hormones are a derivative of cholesterol), and prostaglandins. Eighty per cent of the white matter of the brain is made from essential fatty acids; and nerves have an insulating coat, called the myelin sheath, also composed of the same fatty acids. Hence the saying 'fish is good for your brain' is based on fact.

There are many different fatty acids, but they are divided broadly into two groups, called saturated and unsaturated.

The *saturated fats* tend to be hard, are found in meat, lard, cheese, butter, hardened margarines and overheated oils.

The *unsaturated fats* tend to be liquid or soft at normal temperatures. When unsaturated fats (e.g. vegetable oil) are heated they take on hydrogen atoms and become saturated, hence lose their value.

'Saturated' refers to the number of hydrogen atoms stuck on to the chain of carbon in the fatty acid molecule.

It is the *imbalance* of too much saturated fat in relation to unsaturated that leads to deposition of excess cholesterol, which the liver makes from fats, inside blood vessel walls; this causes heart disease, blood pressure, strokes, etc. Eskimos living on their natural diet which is very high in fish oil are renowned for their lack of the diseases of Western societies, in spite of a high level of total fats in their diet and a large amount of obesity. They are protected because of all the unsaturated fats in fish oils.

Processed vegetable oils and hardened margarines are actually worse for you than butter or cream, because they contain types of saturated fatty acids which block the body's utilization of the good essential fats. Not all polyunsaturated fats (PUFAs) are essential fatty acids. The important essential fatty acids (EFAs) are linoleic acid, linolenic acid and those derived from fish oils.

So why all this emphasis on EFAs in ME?

Essential fatty acids are needed to make, among other things, *prostaglandins*, which have very important functions. There are numerous types of prostaglandins, their function is in regulating the biochemistry and enzyme activities of all body cells. They are very active, but very short-lived.

They are divided into three groups: PG 1, PG 2, PG 3. Within each group are many further types, with different letters, A, B, D, E, F, etc. New prostaglandins are continually being discovered.

A prostaglandin, *PG E 1*, is a product of linoleic acid, an essential fatty acid that has to be obtained from food.

PG E 1 functions

- stops platelets sticking together
- * improves circulation by dilating small blood vessels
- lowers blood pressure
- * restores normal shape and movement of red blood cells
- inhibits inflammation
- lowers cholesterol production
- enhances effects of insulin
- inhibits multiplication of cancer cells
- * activates T lymphocytes in immune system
- * has effects on transmission at nerve endings and nerve condition

(* means relevant in ME)

PG E 1 is found to be low in diabetics, in those with hardening of the arteries, in many psychiatric disorders, and in *allergic people*.

There are various things which may block the synthesis of PG E 1. Let us look at the pathway from linoleic acid to PG E 1, and see what things block it, and what other factors are needed:

(1) *Linoleic acid* (in pure vegetable oils, nuts, seeds)
needs: zinc, magnesium, biotin, vitamin B_6
blocked by: excess saturated fats, alcohol, diabetes, ageing, chemicals, cortisol, and *viral infections*
↓
(2) *Gamma-linolenic acid* (GLA) (in evening primrose oil)
↓ needs vitamin B_6
(3) *Dihomo-gamma-linolenic acid* (DGLA)
↓ needs vitamin C and vitamin B_3
(4) *Prostaglandin E 1*

Note that the block in the pathway from linoleic acid to PG E 1 can be bypassed if *GLA* is supplied in the diet – the GLA that occurs naturally in certain seeds, especially the seeds of the evening primrose and blackcurrants, the main sources of commercially prepared GLA supplements.

So from knowing that PG E 1 synthesis is inhibited by viral infections, it can be understood why in a chronic viral infection one may develop many symptoms due to lack of PG E 1, especially *allergies*.

Linoleic acid makes another prostaglandin called PG E 2, via arachidonic acid, which also occurs in meat.

PG 2 series have different actions from PG 1:

They make smooth muscle contract and promote platelet stickiness – platelets are the tiny cells in the blood that form clots. They also produce inflammation, reddening of skin, and swelling.

Arachidonic acid, a product of linoleic acid, itself leads to inflammation, and also occurs in meat. So if a diet is high in arachidonic acid (meat) but low in linoleic acid (vegetables) there will tend to be greater production of the pro-inflammatory PG 2 series and less of the anti-inflammatory PG 1 series. A diet with a greater amount of vegetables and fish relative to meat will tend to produce relatively more of the PG E 1 prostaglandins, hence less inflammation, allergies or clotting.

PG 3 series

Prostaglandin group 3 series and related substances are formed from alpha linolenic acid, found in beans, wheat and spinach, and from eicosapentanoeic acid (EPA) found mainly in fish oils. The PG 3 series are important in prevention of thrombosis.

It is currently thought that a combination of essential fatty acids from vegetable oils, nuts and seeds, and those in fish oils, is best for health.

This can be achieved by eating generous amounts of a wide range of vegetables, that includes green leafy vegetable daily; having about four teaspoons daily of pure unrefined vegetable oil (cold pressed olive oil is best) on salads in dressing; using a high quality unsaturated margarine; avoiding oil used for deep frying (better to use a little olive oil for occasional frying); eating fish two or three times a week. The best fish are herring, mackerel, sardine, tuna, whitebait, shellfish, and roe.

Some people may need to take supplements of EFAs, primarily of gamma-linolenic acid (GLA), which is marketed as oil of evening primrose or blackcurrant seed oil. This is recommended for ME sufferers, especially if they have become allergic.

Fluids

Many people are horrified at the idea of abandoning most of their usual beverages. In an average day, a person may drink four cups of coffee, three cups of tea, a glass or two of wine or a pint of beer, and perhaps a bottle or can of some sweet fizzy concoction if the weather is warm. All these might contain a total of eight to 10 or more teaspoons of sugar for some people!

What is wrong with water? Most people rarely drink it, and the chemical chlorinated taste of most brands of tap-water is certainly off-putting. Water tastes better if it is spring water, or filtered, and some people may prefer to remove chlorine, lead, copper, nitrates, etc., from drinking water by using a domestic filter. An average person needs to drink at least two pints of water a day in one form or another, in addition to fluid in food – and more in hot weather or if ill. During a relapse or period of severe illness it is advisable to increase the fluid intake to four pints a day or more by drinking warm water between meals. This will help the kidneys to flush out toxins and other products of the body's reaction to the virus.

Many ME people have digestive problems, due to lack of digestive enzymes and stomach acid. If you drink fluids with, or just after your meal, the digestive juices are diluted and digestion is weakened. It is better to drink fluids between main meals, i.e. at least half an hour before or two hours after.

The best drinks are water, diluted pure fruit juices (undiluted they contain too much fruit sugar), herbal teas; tea if you want it should be weak, and of low caffeine level such as china tea. If you must have coffee, then one cup of not very strong ground coffee is better than several cups of instant. Instant and decaffeinated powders are rather chemicalized in their production.

Fibre

Fibre is the indigestible residue (celluloses, pectins, gums and mucilages) composed of cell walls in plant foods, which passes right through the intestines and forms part of the faeces. It has no nutritional value of itself, but it is essential to provide bulk in the large intestine (colon). Its chief property is an absorption of water, making a bulky stool which passes more quickly and smoothly through the colon to the rectum for evacuation.

Lack of fibre may result in:

- Constipation. Besides being uncomfortable, constipation contributes to piles, varicose veins, and undesirable effects of food residues remaining too long in the colon – fermentation, absorption of toxins, etc.
- Diverticulitis
- A higher risk of cancer of the colon
- Too high cholesterol (hence risk of heart disease)
- Gallstones
- Alteration in balance of the bacteria in the colon, which may favour overgrowth of undesirable bugs, such as candida (see Chapter 9). This imbalance is called *dysbiosis*, and may be implicated in many other illnesses.

In spite of much publicity, wheat bran is not the best source of fibre. It may cause problems – bloating, gas, pain, spastic colon – in people who are wheat intolerant, which includes many ME sufferers. Wheat fibre is high in phytates, which combine with calcium, iron, zinc and magnesium to form phytate salts which pass through. Hence absorption of these essential minerals may be impaired. This phytate is only a problem in added wheat bran or in unleavened bread, and is broken down in the leavening process of normal bread.

Iron deficiency is more common in vegetarians who eat a lot of cereal fibre, because of low iron in the diet and prevention of iron absorption by phytates.

The best sources of fibre are from a high intake of mixed fruits and vegetables, wholegrains including oats and unrefined rice rather than just wheat, and some pulses.

You will see from reading this chapter so far that no mention has been made of special or restricted diets. In later chapters, advice will be given about anti-candida and allergy diets.

To summarize, here are the guidelines for a basic healthy diet:

Include	*Avoid if possible*
Complex carbohydrates (wholegrains, brown rice)	Additives, colourings
Fish	Sugar, refined starches
Lean meat, poultry, game, organ meats (liver, etc.)	Alcohol, cola, caffeine
Eggs (free-range), milk, low fat cheese, yoghourt	Processed meats
Lots of fresh vegetables, mixed salad once or twice daily	Foods high in animal fat
Nuts and seeds (e.g. in muesli)	Tinned fruit
Potatoes in skins	Pastry, fried food
Fresh fruit	
Pulses in moderation (if tolerated)	
Pure vegetable oils	

Use fresh ingredients where possible, and organically reared meat if obtainable. Wash all vegetables well. Eat regular meals, maybe four or five small meals a day if there is any tendency to low blood sugar – see Chapter 13.

Do not spend valuable energy travelling long distances to buy organic food, unless you have a freezer to make a bulk buy of meat worthwhile.

In an ideal situation, it would be best for all ME people (and indeed the whole population) to eat food that is 100 per cent free from chemicals.

Get it if you can, or find a neighbour or relative with a vegetable garden, but do not worry unduly about produce from your nearest and easiest shops or supermarkets. There is a greater awareness now about the hazards of chemicals, many supermarkets label foods that are 'organically' produced, and it is worth asking the retailers if they can obtain chemical-free foodstuffs.

However some organic vegetable produce is very expensive and may not be very fresh, and mouldy food is even worse than 'non-organic' fresh stuff, because of the association of ME with yeast infections.

Suggested Further Reading

Let's Get Well, by Adelle Davis (Allen & Unwin, 1983).
Nutritional Medicine, by Stephen Davies and Alan Stewart (Pan, 1987).
Raw Energy, by Leslie and Susannah Kenton (Arrow, 1987).

8

Nutritional Supplements

This is a controversial subject. Some argue that if you eat a well balanced diet of good fresh foods, then it should not be necessary to take extra vitamins or minerals. For someone in perfect health this is probably true.

However, the 'Recommended Daily Allowance' (RDA) for each nutrient is calculated for the average adult of average weight in health, and is frequently the amount which is just sufficient to prevent a deficiency disease. This may be very much less than the amount required by an individual for optimum health and, in disease states, the body's requirements may increase dramatically to a level which cannot be obtained from a normal diet.

Many ME patients have problems with digestion and absorption of food. Signs suggesting this are:

- Weight loss in spite of good food intake
- Stools that contain undigested food
- Stools that float
- Diarrhoea, distension, abdominal pains.

If you have these symptoms, especially weight loss with a good appetite, assume that you are not getting the full value from what you eat. As well as losing protein and fats, you may be losing calcium, iron, zinc, folic acid, vitamin B_{12}, and the fat soluble vitamins A, E and D. Another possible cause of poor intake of nutrients is lack of appetite or nausea.

Possible causes of poor absorption in ME:

(1) Virus infections may cause flattening of the microvilli (tiny projections) on the surface of cells lining the small intestine, hence loss of absorptive surface.
(2) If the pancreas has been involved in a present or earlier virus infection, there may be reduced production of pancreatic digestive enzymes and of bicarbonate which is needed to make the small intestine alkaline.
(3) There may be overactivity of the gut in general, leading to 'intestinal hurry', the food being rushed through the small bowel with insufficient time there for digestion and absorption. This overactivity results from disordered control of the autonomic nervous system.

The other good reason for supplementing a good diet, which should be organized before getting supplements, is to provide as much as possible of the nutrients which are essential for the body's immune system, nervous system and the various glandular functions.

If someone develops ME after a seemingly innocuous viral infection, which is the common onset, then there are likely to be deficiencies of some vital nutrients, from years or perhaps a lifetime of deficiencies in the diet, or even prenatally from poor maternal health, or resulting from earlier infections.

So it seems logical to take whatever is necessary to restore the body to health. It is certainly more logical and safer to correct nutritional imbalances, than to swallow drugs which only modify the symptoms instead of treating the underlying cause of illness.

A big consideration for many ME sufferers who are

trying to decide about supplements is cost. Some can be obtained on prescription, if your GP can be persuaded that this is a worthwhile course to pursue. Otherwise, it helps to work out how much the supplements are going to cost per day, having bought a two months' supply or so, this being the painful part of the purse!

There may be less important things you could give up to pay for improved health, for the time being. For example, the cost of weekly newspapers may be as much as the cost of vitamins and minerals, but not so essential.

Like a lot of decisions with ME, it is a matter of deciding on priorities.

Digestive Enzymes

If you or your doctor think you have poor absorption of food due to lack of digestive enzymes, then taking a preparation of these makes sense. They are obtainable on prescription, and are all made from pancreatic extract, with various trade names, e.g. Pancrex, Nutrizyme. The preparation may be in granules or powder, and should be taken immediately before or with a meal, as it is inactivated by stomach acid.

Hydrochloric acid

The stomach normally secretes digestive juices containing hydrochloric acid in response to and in anticipation of food. In allergic people, chronic viral illness, fevers, diabetes and rheumatoid arthritis, there is frequently achlorhydria, i.e. lack of gastric acid.

This may lead to fermentation in the stomach, bad

breath, gas, and indigestion, especially of protein. The enzyme pepsin needs acidity to work properly to start breaking down protein. Acidity is also needed to absorb calcium and iron.

Hydrochloric acid can be taken in various preparations, on prescription, starting with a small dose with meals (but *not* by those with proven overacidity or symptoms of an ulcer, so consult your doctor first).

Vitamin C

This is one of the most essential vitamins to help you with ME. It cannot be stored in the body, and is needed daily in food.

What does vitamin C do?

(1) Vitamin C is needed to make collagen, the fibrous framework of most of the body. It is vital for the continuous repair and regeneration of body tissues.
(2) Vitamin C is used by the adrenal gland to make the hormones noradrenaline and cortisol. The adrenal gland in health is rich in ascorbic acid.
(3) Vitamin C is a powerful anti-oxidant, it mops up 'free radicals' of oxygen which are released in various biochemical reactions, and which may cause cell damage.
(4) Vitamin C has important effects on the *immune system*:
    (a) It promotes
    - formation of lymphocytes;
    - lymphocyte mobility;
    - white cell ability to engulf other material (phagocytosis). Phagocytic white cells can

only consume bacteria and dead cells if they contain ascorbic acid, which is vitamin C.

(b) It is involved in the manufacture of antibodies (immunoglobulins) and is needed to make one of the chemicals used in immune reactions, called complement.

In 1972, Irvine Stone described vitamin C and infections:

- it kills or slows down growth of bacteria;
- it detoxicates and renders harmless bacterial toxins;
- it maintains phagocytosis;
- it is non-toxic and can be administered in large doses.

In 1979, at the National Cancer Institute of USA, an investigation found that giving 5 grams vitamin C per day to healthy people aged 18–30 led to doubling their rate of formation of new lymphocytes.

An increased intake of vitamin C leads to greater production of interferon. Interferons are proteins with anti viral activity, produced by virus infected cells. They spread to non-infected cells and help them resist infection.

Vitamin C inhibits the synthesis of inflammatory prostaglandins (the PG E 2 ones), therefore is anti-inflammatory.

Much valuable work on the use of high dose vitamin C to treat infections, cancer, and many disorders of immunity such as rheumatoid arthritis, has been done by Dr Linus Pauling. While many sceptics have dismissed his findings, Dr Pauling argued that in tests where people took vitamin C and no benefit was found, they did not take a large enough dose. The

RDA of vitamin C in Britain is 30 mg (obtained from half an orange!), but a more realistic minimum amount for good health would be 100 mg.

Much of Dr Pauling's reasoning for a greatly increased need of vitamin C comes from his calculations of the amounts of various nutrients in the diet of our ancestors. As man evolved he was unable to make vitamin C in the body, unlike most other mammals, so he would have survived by having the optimum amount in his daily food. If you estimate the amount of food a hunter–gatherer would have needed each day to keep him healthy, it would contain about 3 grams of vitamin C – a hundred times the modern 'daily allowance'. Early man's diet had a much greater ratio of raw fruits, vegetables, nuts and berries than that of a twentieth-century Western diet. (However, his total food intake was not usually enough for health.)

A person with an infection, or under stress such as major surgery, or severe emotional shock, needs far more; vitamin C is used up by the adrenal glands in response to stress, wound healing requires extra vitamin C, and it is used by the immune system to fight infection.

Vitamin C cannot be stored in the body, and any that is not used is excreted in the urine. The chief undesirable effect from taking more than is needed is diarrhoea. This is why the term 'bowel tolerance' is used when advising people how much to take.

It is suggested that you take vitamin C in divided doses rather than one large dose, and start with 1 gram daily, 500 mg morning and evening. Increase this by 1 gram daily, until you have loose bowel motions, then cut it back to 1 gram less. This may work out at anything from 3 grams to 12 grams a day. ME sufferers who claim that vitamin C made no difference to them are usually taking too little to have any immune stimulating effect. People with a history of kidney stones need a smaller dose, no more than 1 gram daily, in divided doses and with plenty of water.

Pure vitamin C is ascorbic acid, a weak acid, but still an acid. The cheapest way to get it is as pure ascorbic acid powder from a supplier. One level teaspoon of powder is about 3 grams. It should be completely dissolved in water or fruit juice, and taken with or just after food to avoid irritating the stomach, which does not usually happen. To 'buffer' the acidity, a little bicarbonate of soda can be added. (For suppliers, see Appendix A.)

The next best vitamin C is the buffered 1 gram tablets (e.g. Redoxan) which dissolve to make a fizzy drink. If you stay at 1 or 2 grams a day, this is fine; above that it becomes expensive.

Some ME patients take 1 to 3 grams a day when in a stable state, and increase if exposed to infection or at the start of a relapse.

Vitamin B_6 (Pyridoxine)

Vitamin B_6 is important in many chemical processes.

It is needed in the metabolism of protein and amino acids. It is involved in the production and reactions of many body chemicals, including those which affect mood and behaviour.

It is involved in sugar metabolism, also in pathways of essential fatty acids (EFAs), which are needed for the immune system; vitamin B_6 is needed for some minerals to work, especially magnesium.

Deficiency signs are: depression, irritability, red, greasy, scaly skin on the face. However, a lack of vitamin B_6 alone is unusual, there is usually a multiple B vitamin deficiency.

Recommended supplement level is 20–50 mg daily, as part of a B-complex preparation.

All the B vitamins work and interact together, so *individual B supplements are not recommended*.

Vitamin B_{12}

This is only required in small amounts daily, about 1 microgram. It is found in meat, fish, and eggs; vegans risk a deficiency of it. As it is absorbed in the small intestine and needs a substance secreted by the stomach to combine with before absorption, people with deficient stomach juice or malabsorption in the small intestine are at risk from B_{12} deficiency.

Vitamin B_{12} is concerned with red cell production, and with nervous system functions. A lack of it can lead to anaemia, abnormal fatigue, pins and needles in feet, stumbling gait, and mental confusion.

It is worthwhile for chronic ME sufferers to have their blood B_{12} level checked, especially if these neurological symptoms are prominent, if there are digestive/absorption problems, and if the person is middle aged or elderly. With the current publicity about ME, there may well be people who think they have ME, especially in the older age group, who in fact have vitamin B_{12} deficiency.

If there is a deficiency, supplementation is best given by injection, 1 mg every one to three months. Some ME sufferers do report an improvement from B_{12} injections, although no clinical trials have yet been done.

Orally, B_{12} is taken as part of a B complex, but this is not appropriate for someone with lack of stomach acid.

A good vitamin B complex should be yeast free (because many ME patients have a candida–yeast problem), and contain all the B vitamins as follows:

- Thiamine B_1 } these should be about the same amount, 20–50 mg
- Riboflavin B_2 }
- Pyridoxine B_6 }
- Niacin B_3
- Pantothenate B_5
- Cyanocobalamin B_{12}
- Folic acid
- Para Amino Benzoic Acid (PABA)
- Biotin.

Vitamin A

Vitamin A itself occurs in animal produce; the best sources are animal and fish livers, kidneys, eggs and milk products. Beta-carotene, a precursor of vitamin A, is obtained from vegetables, particularly carrots, and other green, yellow or orange coloured plants.

Vitamin A deficiency is one of the commonest causes of blindness in poor countries, because of poor diet, especially in small children.

It is important for maintaining mucous membranes, skin, and cell membranes.

It is needed for resistance to infections. Vitamin A is one of the 'anti-oxidants' (along with vitamins C, E and selenium), therefore prevents damage to cell membranes, and has an important role in cancer prevention.

As it is fat soluble, and stored in the body, very high doses can accumulate and cause toxicity. Doses of up to 20,000 units daily are safe, but 7,000 to 15,000 units a day are sufficient unless there are particular indications of deficiency. The best way to supplement vitamin A is as part of a balanced multi-vitamin preparation, or in fish liver oil capsules, which also provide valuable essential fatty acids.

Pantothenic Acid (Vitamin B_5)

This little known vitamin is one of the B family. It occurs widely in many foods; it is essential for the proper function of adrenal glands and for making antibodies. It is one of the anti-stress vitamins and is important for fighting infection and allergies.

It is present in most B complex preparations. It seems to be helpful in high doses in stress-related diseases, and conditions where the immune system is not working properly such as allergies and rheumatoid arthritis. It is recommended for ME, and can be taken as calcium pantothenate in doses of 300 up to 1,000 mg.

The symptoms of pantothenic acid deficiency (produced in volunteers) are remarkably similar to those of ME, and of multiple allergies. It has even been suggested that members of families who are all allergic may have some inherited factor which greatly increases the need for this vitamin.

Vitamin E

This is another fat soluble vitamin, and most important for its anti-oxidant properties (like A, C and selenium). It occurs in vegetables, nuts and eggs, and recommended supplement is 100 to 200 IU daily.

What do anti-oxidants do?

Oxygen is essential for cells to live. However, in certain circumstances it produces toxic oxygen derivatives which can combine with other molecules and cause damage to cells and alter their function, or cause them to become cancerous, or to die. These nasty oxygen products are called 'free radicals', and are mopped up and made safe by anti-oxidants. Anti-oxidants are vitamins A, C and E, and various enzymes which contain trace elements such as selenium, zinc, manganese, and copper. The 'free radicals' cause damage to the fatty acid part of cell walls.

Free radicals have multiple sources, including chemicals in air pollution and food, and cigarette smoke, but are also produced by lymphocytes in inflammation, e.g. killing virus infected cells.

In ME, there seems to be a persistent low grade viral infection, and disordered cell functions all over the body. Some doctors have used the term 'sick cell syndrome' about ME. So it seems logical to minimize damage to the cells from 'free radical' oxygen products, by ensuring a good intake of nutrients needed for a good anti-oxidant system.

Zinc

Zinc is a trace element which is necessary for a wide range of chemical reactions in the body. Studies of zinc and its many roles have begun relatively recently, and there is still much to discover.

What is zinc needed for?

- For all growth
- For wound healing and all tissue repair

- For maturation and function of sexual organs
- For normal development of the unborn child
- For the immune system
- For the normal function of all the senses: vision, taste, smell and sight
- For normal hair growth
- For normal muscle function
- For mental functions: emotional functions, intelligence, appetite, sleep patterns
- For protein metabolism
- For conversion of essential fatty acids to prostaglandins (see pages 98–100).

Some results of zinc deficiency

- Impaired wound healing
- Loss of sense of taste or smell
- Slow growth
- Infertility
- Hair loss
- Skin problems (including acne)
- *Allergies*
- *Poor resistance to infection*
- White spots on finger nails
- *Depression and other mental disturbances.*

Causes of risk of zinc deficiency

- Poor intake – vegan diet, slimming diets, strict allergy diets, poor appetite, the elderly, alcoholics, people on special synthetic diets or intravenous feeding
- Poor absorption – high fibre diet with lots of bran
- Iron tablets
- Alcoholic liver disease
- Low stomach acid

- Lack of pancreatic enzymes
- Malabsorption due to gluten sensitivity (coeliac disease).

In theory, a balanced diet should provide enough zinc. The daily requirement is about 15 mg for a healthy adult – more in pregnancy, much more after major surgery, burns, or any severe stress.

The assessment of zinc status is at present not very satisfactory. Levels estimated in blood plasma, urine or hair do not seem to be accurate. The blood level can vary enormously throughout twenty-four hours. The most reliable method is by analysis of sweat, but this requires specialist apparatus.

Since in ME there is evidence of a persistent virus, of disordered immune function, and in many there may be problems with digestion and absorption of food, it is sensible to take extra zinc. A zinc supplement is best taken apart from food, since its absorption is inhibited by iron and various foods.

A preparation giving 20–50 mg elemental zinc, as zinc ororate, zinc sulphate, or amino chelated zinc, can be taken at bedtime, with no ill effects.

Therapists with access to accurate assessment of zinc levels say that every ME patient that they see is low in zinc.

Magnesium

Everyone knows how important calcium is, because it is one of the main constituents of the skeleton, but magnesium is not so well known.

Magnesium is absolutely vital for normal cell function; it is present inside every single living cell as well as in teeth and bones. The correct balance of calcium and magnesium across cell membranes is essential for transmission of nerve impulses, and for muscle contraction and relaxation.

Magnesium is also involved in many enzyme systems and chemical reactions in the body.

Magnesium occurs naturally in hard tap-water, in whole grains, green vegetables, nuts and beans.

A deficiency is most likely in someone on a poor diet, and living in a soft water area.

Magnesium deficiency leads to:

- Many neurological symptoms
- Muscle cramps or twitching
- Heart rhythm abnormalities
- Tingling and numbness
- Muscle inco-ordination
- Overactivity
- Mental confusion
- Depression
- Muscular weakness.

Magnesium is needed for the body to use vitamins B_6, B_1, and EFAs.

In ME, there appears to be a delay in recovery of muscle fibres after contracting, the result of disordered muscle cell functioning. A low level of magnesium in the cell may contribute to this.

Supplementation is advisable for this reason, and to ensure proper utilization of EFAs and B vitamins. Symptoms of constipation, insomnia, irritability and muscle fatigue may improve on taking extra magnesium.

A daily intake of 200–300 mg is enough, in various preparations. Magnesium is available together with calcium in dolomite tablets, in a ratio of 2:1

calcium : magnesium, which is a good balance. Some nutritional experts advise that they should be taken as separate preparations because of possible contamination of dolomite. If some or all of the magnesium is taken in the evening, it may help with insomnia and 'jumping muscles' at night.

As well as zinc, magnesium is the most important mineral to take for ME.

Iron

Iron deficiency is commoner than is at first apparent from doing blood tests. It is possible to have a low body iron content before a blood test shows anaemia.

Those most at risk from iron deficiency are:

- Women who are menstruating, especially if the periods are heavy
- Pregnant women
- Strict vegetarians
- People on a poor diet through poverty or ignorance
- People with malabsorption, and with low stomach acid production
- Those with poor appetite, anorexia nervosa
- Children on a poor diet.

Iron is not only needed to make haemoglobin, which carries oxygen to all tissues in red blood cells, but for many enzyme reactions.

Symptoms of iron deficiency:

- Fatigue, breathlessness and thumping heart on exertion

- Pallor, pale concave nails
- Maybe difficulty with swallowing, sore tongue.

The best natural sources of iron are organ meats such as liver, red meats, egg yolks, legumes, molasses, parsley, shellfish, wholegrains, nuts and green vegetables.

Absorption of iron is impaired by wholegrains, tea and coffee, and is helped by vitamin C. So it is a good thing to have salad and/or fresh fruit with main meals.

Unless you have a low serum iron level it is probably not necessary to take a separate iron supplement. The average amount in a good multi-mineral supplement is about 20mg. If a higher level is needed, then ferrous gluconate 200 mg a day can be taken, not at the same time as a zinc supplement. Overt iron deficiency is not commonly found in ME patients, but is important to exclude if there is evidence of poor absorption, pallor and shortness of breath.

Selenium

This mineral occurs widely in food, and its functions in man are not yet fully understood. The important role of selenium which has been researched is as an anti-oxidant, mopping up 'free radicals', and thus it helps protect cells from damage, ageing and cancerous changes.

The relevance of selenium to ME is that many allergies develop, there is frequently sensitivity to chemicals, and muscle and brain cells do not function properly. A theory linking all these is of poor oxidation mechanisms, and the presence of those nasty free radicals.

Some ME patients with severe chemical allergies

have improved on a regime which includes all the anti-oxidants, vitamins A, C, E and selenium.

Selenium is toxic in high doses. A supplement of 100 to 200 micrograms per day should not be exceeded.

Essential Fatty Acid Supplements

The important role of EFAs was discussed in Chapter 7. If one is getting EFAs in pure vegetable oils, vegetables, nuts and fish in a good diet, why is there any need for supplements?

Remember the pathway from linoleic acid to prostaglandin E 1 (the anti-inflammatory PG which boosts lymphocyte function, discussed on page 98):

> The conversion of linoleic acid to gamma-linolenic acid (GLA) can be blocked by several things, including *viral infections*, lack of vitamin B_6, zinc, magnesium and excess animal fats.
>
> EFA supplementation using GLA in evening primrose oil bypasses these blocks, and the GLA can go straight on in the pathway to form prostaglandin E1.

EFAs and their products are needed to make cell membranes, and are important constituents of white matter in nervous tissue. EFA supplements are used with success to help patients who have multiple sclerosis. MS is a disease of myelin tissue, but defects in cell membranes have been discovered, and present evidence suggests that the underlying problem is an inability to handle fats properly. Some speculate that a virus infection may be implicated.

A neurologist, Professor E. J. Field, has treated

many MS patients with evening primrose oil. Those in the early stages of the illness seem to respond best.

He has also seen many ME sufferers over the years; some symptoms are common to both conditions, and not infrequently someone labelled as multiple sclerosis turns out to have ME. Professor Field prescribes evening primrose oil to his ME patients, and estimates that about two-thirds of them have some improvement.

As yet, there have been no medical trials on the value of supplementing GLA to ME patients. But for all the above reasons it is recommended, and certainly will do no harm.

Suitable dosage is at least 1500 mg daily of gamma oil from whatever source; some doctors suggest 3000 mg daily – that is, from three to six 500 mg capsules daily. Vitamin E should always be taken with GLA, and is included in some preparations.

It is not clear whether fish oils should be taken as well. They seem to be of value in rheumatoid arthritis and heart disease. If no fish is eaten in the diet, then fish oils as cod liver oil capsules, or a preparation such as Max EPA, three to six capsules can be taken.

EFAs work best when there is enough zinc, magnesium, vitamins C and E, and vitamin B_6.

Amino Acids

Amino acids are the basic building blocks for the manufacture of all proteins in the body, including antibodies, all the lymphokines produced by white cells, digestive enzymes, neuro-transmitters and hormones. Without these building blocks, taking vitamin and mineral supplements may be a waste of money. Certain amino acids are known to be needed for proper brain function, and tryptophan and phenylalanine can improve mood.

Unless you can have a full analysis of amino acid levels in your body carried out, you will not know which, if any, to take. Anyone with ME who has symptoms which suggest poor absorption would be as well taking a supplement of 'free form' amino acids. These are available either on prescription or as capsules in a health food shop, and should be taken between meals with some water three times a day.

I know of a number of ME people who did not improve with a very nutritious diet, plus supplements, but felt an increase in strength and clearing of the mind after starting to take free form amino acids, myself included.

Summary of Supplements

Ideally, someone considering taking nutritional supplements should consult a physician or biochemist who specializes in nutrition, and have his or her individual nutritional needs worked out. This is not usually possible, due to distances and the cost of a consultation and tests. If you have such an expert near you, one who uses reliable methods to assess levels of nutrients, I do recommend at least one consultation, which may save you taking some things that are not necessary.

Failing the chance of such advice, then a suitable 'package' of supplements for someone with ME would be:

- A good quality multi-vitamin and mineral tablet daily – ideally one which has high levels of B vitamins, and is yeast free

- Evening primrose oil or equivalent 1 to 3 gm daily
- Zinc 20–50 mg at night
- Magnesium 200–300 mg daily
- Selenium 100–200 micrograms daily
- Vitamin E 100–200 IU daily
- Calcium pantothenate 300 mg daily (up to 1,000 mg a day if very stressed or if badly allergic)
- Vitamin C minimum 1 gm a day, preferably 3 gm, rising to 9 gm or more if very unwell or exposed to infection
- Free form amino acids 5–20 mg daily.

There is no benefit to be gained, but possibly some harm and certainly loss of money, in exceeding these doses without medical supervision!

Pancreatic enzymes, hydrochloric acid, and amino acids as appropriate, are helpful particularly for those ME sufferers with marked digestive symptoms and evidence of poor absorption.

Two other substances are suggested for ME by some therapists. These are:

- Germanium, a mineral needed in trace amounts;
- Coenzyme Q, an enzyme involved in energy production.

In theory taking these should improve energy levels. However they are expensive, and I have not found any evidence that they are particularly useful in ME. They certainly would be of no use if other essential things like magnesium, zinc and B vitamins were deficient.

If you want to try them, and can afford them, they will not do any harm. But I cannot promise at this present time that they will do any good. More information about these substances may become available in the next few years.

Suggested Further Reading

The Vitamin Bible, by Earl Mindell (Arlington, 1984).
Evening Primrose Oil, by Judy Graham (Thorsons, 1984).
The Amino Revolution, by Robert Erdman and Meiron Jones (Century, 1987).

9

Candida Albicans

At least two-thirds of ME sufferers have their condition made worse by an infection with the yeast called candida. This is a controversial subject, and there are various schools of thought. At one extreme are people who claim that candida is the number one culprit in all ME patients, and that if you can get rid of it you will be a great deal better or cured. At the other end are those who cannot accept that candida infection has anything whatsoever to do with ME, or indeed any ill health, and that trying to treat it is a waste of time.

A lot of people have now heard the word candida, but for those who have not, Candida Albicans is one of the many bugs which is to be found living in and on all of us. It is a fungus, one of the yeast family of organisms, and is best known for causing thrush in the mouth in babies, giving sore white moist plaques in the mouth and on the tongue, and thrush in the vagina of women (which is where the babies pick it up during birth). It can also cause nappy rash on babies, soreness and itching around the anus in adults, and infection of the skin of the genitals in men. Candida also lives in small numbers in our guts, and on the skin especially in warm moist areas. In a healthy person with a strong defence system, candida keeps its place and does not cause any symptoms. It is so prevalent that at least 90 per cent of children have had exposure to it at six months old, evidenced by finding a reaction on skin testing.

The most extreme cases of candida yeast multiplying and invading all parts of the body, including the bloodstream and the lungs and brain, are in very ill people whose immune systems have completely stopped working. These include leukaemias, people with immuno-suppressive treatment, some overwhelming infections which wipe out the bone marrow, and AIDS, where the T lymphocytes are all knocked out.

It must be emphasized again that the mild disorder in the immune system that appears to be part of the ME syndrome is **quite different** to the total collapse of immunity seen in the above examples!

Candida is only one of a huge variety of yeasts, moulds, viruses, and bacteria which live on, in and around us. The large bowel, or colon, contains several pounds in weight of bacteria, most of which are actually necessary for manufacture of some vitamins, fermentation of undigested food remains, and breakdown of mucus. They stay in their place because of the colon wall, and white blood cells and antibodies circulating in the local blood vessels mop up any stray bugs that try and move into the rest of the body. Similarly, an immune system's surveillance takes care that these 'commensal' (meaning living with) bugs, that live on skin in various places, in genital areas, and in the mouth, should stay put and in small numbers.

There are some circumstances which allow candida to multiply and cause trouble.

Factors that Favour Candida Growth

- *Warmth and moisture.*
- *Sugar* – e.g. diabetics, and too much sugar in diet. Just remember how bread rises with yeast and

sugar, and how much sugar is needed to ferment beer or wine.

- *A weakened defence system* – such as in ME, poor nutrition, chronic infections.
- *Altered hormone levels* – contraceptive pill, pregnancy, taking steroid drugs (cortisone, prednisolone).
- *Taking broad spectrum antibiotics* – because these not only kill off the bacteria which are making you ill, such as with tonsillitis or bladder infection, but they destroy large numbers of the friendly bacteria in the colon. This results in a relative 'overgrowth' of yeasts, which are left unharmed by antibiotics. The imbalance of microbes thus created is known as *dysbiosis* – i.e. a disharmony of bugs. Dysbiosis may underlie many conditions of ill health, including ME. The problem with antibiotics may not be so bad with a short five- to seven-day course of a selective one such as penicillin, which only kills a narrow range of bugs such as those causing septic throats or infected gums. It is the broad spectrum antibiotics, designed to 'kill all known germs', such as tetracycline and ampicillin, which lead to dysbiosis, especially if given repeatedly or over a period of time.

Two conditions when long-term broad spectrum antibiotics tend to be given are the skin condition acne, and recurrent cystitis (bladder infection). It is unfortunate that these problems may actually be caused by a candida infection, and made worse by antibiotics.

Another source of long-term antibiotics may be from meat and poultry fed on foodstuffs to which antibiotics have been added, to prevent disease in intensively reared animals. The quantity is of course small, but must have some effect on our finely balanced colonies of bugs over a period of time.

Let us not ignore the fact that antibiotics have saved thousands of lives. Pneumonia used to be capable of killing young people within five days, before the advent of penicillin. Infection and gangrene killed many thousands in the First World War. It is just unfortunate that in the last two decades there has been a tendency to overprescribe broad spectrum antibiotics, often as an umbrella tactic, instead of encouraging the body to overcome what may be quite a minor localized infection; or often a virus infection which is not touched by antibiotics anyway. So a generation has grown up who may have had antibiotics many times in childhood for ear or throat infections, in adolescence for spots, and as young adults for bouts of flu or bladder infections.

Given favourable conditions, candida can proliferate quite fast, and cause *local symptoms*:

> Vaginal thrush, cystitis, infection of prostate gland and male genitals, skin rashes of the groin or armpits, fungal infections of the nails, white patches and ulcers on the gums and mouth, infection of tongue, throat and gullet. These are all surface infections.

More seriously, the yeast can change its shape into a fungal form, with long root structures which enable it to penetrate through mucous membranes of the gut, vagina, or mouth, and enter the bloodstream. It is thought that in this invasive form, called mycelial, candida may produce toxins by its action on fermenting sugar, producing a nasty substance called acetaldehyde. This would explain why the symptoms of a generalized candida infection can resemble those of an alcoholic hangover:

headache, nausea, lack of concentration, irritability, general feeling of being poisoned – as with alcohol.

The change into the invasive form of candida is favoured by a deficiency of biotin, one of the B vitamins. There is some difficulty in knowing what symptoms may be due to candida spread in your body, if you have ME; so many symptoms are the same.

Candida is thought to underlie many conditions, including:

cystitis, prostatitis, endometriosis, irritable bowel syndrome, vaginal discharge, premenstrual tension, depression, rapid mood changes, sudden weight gain, joint pains, muscle aching, fatigue, athlete's foot, acne, sneezing, sore throats, asthma, food allergies, chemical allergies, abdominal bloating, loss of sexual drive.

As you can see, much of this list overlaps with typical ME symptoms. However, there are some clear indications of candida overgrowth.

Candida Assessment Guide

History

(1) Have you been on oral contraceptives for a year or more?
(2) Have you ever had steroids (prednisolone, cortisone, or ACTH (corticotrophin) injections)?
(3) Have you had frequent courses of antibiotics, e.g. four times in one year, or a course lasting six weeks or more?
(4) Have you had long-term antibiotics for acne?

(5) Have you been pregnant?
(6) Have you had immuno-suppressant drugs?

Symptoms

(1) Have you had cystitis, vaginitis, or prostatitis?
(2) Have you had thrush more than once?
(3) Have you ever had fungal infections of nails or skin, e.g. athlete's foot?
(4) Do you have chemical allergies – worse from exposure to tobacco smoke, petrol, perfumes, paints, printer's ink, etc.?
(5) Are your symptoms worse in damp weather or in a damp and mouldy house?
(6) Do you have premenstrual bloating, irritability, or depression?
(7) Do you have bloating after meals, or alternate diarrhoea and constipation?
(8) Are your symptoms worse for eating sweet foods, or alcohol?
(9) Do you *crave* sweets, or alcohol?
(10) Do you have itching or burning in the anus?

If you answer yes to one or more questions in History, and have two or more positive symptoms, then it is likely that candida overgrowth plays some part in your ME illness.

There is no one reliable blood test that can tell you if candida overgrowth is causing your symptoms. However the combination of finding antibodies to candida, together with changes in T lymphocytes in the blood, have been found in most patients with obvious candida-related illness in a study in the USA. Skin testing with diluted candida extract produces a positive result in most of the population, so does not help. Candida can be isolated from the gut of everyone if it is looked for. The best test at present is to treat it and see if symptoms improve.

It is quite possible to have a candida problem without having the obvious symptoms such as thrush. Chemical sensitivity and intolerance to some foods are extremely common. The headaches, irritability, lethargy and lack of concentration that are so common in ME may result from

(a) the virus interfering with brain cells
(b) toxins such as acetaldehyde produced by candida
(c) chemical sensitivity
(d) absorption of larger than usual molecules of partly digested food, particularly proteins.

An explanation of (d) is that the mucous membrane lining of the gut becomes 'leaky', and allows peptides to enter the circulation, which would normally have been broken into amino acids by enzymes in the gut. These peptides, or partially digested proteins, are seen as 'foreign' by the body's immune system, which over-reacts to their presence and leads to allergy symptoms. These food products, commonly from proteins such as milk, gluten from grains, or egg, may themselves act like toxins to the brain, and cause depression, irritability, headache and various other mental symptoms.

Before studying ways of overcoming candida infections, please understand that:

(a) not everyone with ME has a candida problem, although probably at least two-thirds are affected; this estimate is based on a questionnaire study, and is probably an underestimate.
(b) treating candida effectively will make you feel better if there is a problem, and may well clear up

or improve the allergies. There is no guarantee that you will get rid of ME immediately. However, through removing one of the stresses on the immune system the body's natural healing powers will have a better chance of fighting the virus.

(c) if you are going to embark on an anti-candida programme, it is worth giving it a serious trial for about three months at least, rather than being half-hearted about it, then deciding it doesn't help.

There are three divisions of the attack on candida:

(1) modifying the diet to starve it of sugar;
(2) strengthening the body's natural resistance with nutritional supplements;
(3) taking specific anti-candida medication.

The Anti-Candida Diet

The reasons for making changes in how you eat are to deprive candida of its nourishment which is **sugar**, to avoid consuming any other moulds or fungi, and to eat nutritiously to strengthen the natural defences.

Now if you have put into practice the guidelines for healthy eating described in Chapter 7, then you are half-way there. A strict anti-candida diet would also prohibit bread made with yeast, cheese, vinegar, anything else fermented such as soya sauce; it would also restrict carbohydrate intake to 80 gm or so a day. What is more important than restricting carbohydrates is completely to cut out refined carbohydrates, i.e. sugar of all kinds and refined flour, and to eat complex carbohydrates such as brown rice, oats, other wholegrains, potatoes in skins, wholemeal pasta.

If an ME sufferer is already underweight, he or she

must *not* embark on a diet which is going to make them lose even more. It is just as important to feed the patient as to starve the candida.

Another objection to a very strict diet for ME sufferers is that there is enough to contend with if you are ill, without adding to the problems by imposing difficult dietary reforms. A strict anti-candida regime also advises no fruit, because fruit contains fructose, which is a sugar. In practice, a sensible compromise is to have no more than two pieces of fresh fruit a day, and to avoid those high in sugar or which may have yeasts on the skin (e.g. grapes).

It is essential to have enough protein, for reasons of rebuilding a body that is diseased and because the immune system requires all the essential amino acids to make antibodies, enzymes, hormones, etc.

(1) *Foods allowed*

- Potatoes
- Fresh vegetables of all kinds, especially garlic, onion and cabbage family
- Meat, fish, eggs – preferably antibiotic and hormone free
- Wholegrains – brown rice, oats, muesli (no sugar), crispbreads, oatcakes, wholemeal pasta
- Pure vegetable oils
- Milk, butter, live unsweetened yoghourt
- Fresh nuts
- Pulses – lentils, beans (but caution if they give you wind; they must be well cooked)
- Herb teas, water, weak tea.

(2) *Foods to avoid*

- *Sugar* of all kinds – including molasses, honey, brown sugar

- Anything containing sugar – jams, marmalade, sweets, cakes, biscuits, canned drink, some cereals, canned fruit; **read labels**!
- *Alcohol* in all forms – it makes ME and candida patients ill
- Fermented food and drink (but see section on yeasts on page 136), vinegar, ginger ale, soya sauce, tofu, miso, tempeh (all soya derivatives), buttermilk, cheeses – especially blue cheese
- Ready shelled nuts and dried fruit. These often have moulds on the surface, and dried fruit is rich in fruit sugar
- Melon and grapes
- Mushrooms and truffles
- Black tea
- Anything pickled
- Any food which is mouldy, so vegetables and fruit should be as fresh as possible
- Canned or frozen citrus juices.

(3) *Foods allowed in moderation*

- Wholemeal bread – ideally none at all if made with yeast for the first four weeks, then perhaps two medium slices a day if tolerated (if not, it will probably cause bloating and worsening of symptoms)
- Cottage cheese
- Fresh fruit
- Diluted fresh fruit juice (diluted at least two parts water to one part juice) used soon after opening.

On a really strict diet, you would not have anything in category (3), nor any milk or milk products. It is thought that the lactose in milk helps feed candida. If you feel you want to try the strict diet for the first four weeks or so, that is fine, provided you eat enough overall, and do not find the whole exercise too stressful. A lot depends on how you have been eating up till now, your weight, and also on your motivation.

The most important things to avoid are **sugar, alcohol** and **fermented things**.

Note: Until recently, the standard advice given was to avoid eating anything containing yeast, moulds or fungi. Dr William G. Crook, in his book, *The Yeast Connection*, suggests that not all candida patients are affected by other yeasts. He suggests that one should completely cut out all yeast-containing foods for at least a week, then test to see if yeast causes trouble. This can be done by chewing a fragment of a brewer's yeast tablet.

If no symptoms develop after 10 minutes, have another bit, and continue to have pieces of yeast tablet for an hour. If there is no reaction, have another yeast tablet, and if that is all right, then he suggests trying some food such as mushrooms the next day. Of course, if there is any reaction early on in the testing, you should stop and either assume there is a yeast sensitivity, or try again to confirm a few days later.

The point of finding out if other yeasts and moulds affect you is that if they do *not*, then you can eat ordinary bread, have mushrooms sometimes, and the diet is much less arduous to follow. Dr Crook advises that, even if not yeast-sensitive, a person trying to deal with candida should still be moderate in having yeasts and moulds in their diet, and should stop them and retest if the condition gets worse. Another great benefit from finding you are not affected by yeasts is that you can take brewer's yeast tablets as Vitamin B supplements. They are also the best source of chromium, the mineral which is essential for proper blood sugar control.

However, alcohol should still be avoided, whether or not yeasts upset you.

Obviously someone who eats a lot of cakes, biscuits, sweets, cheese, pickles, canned fruit and convenience foods, takes sugar in tea, and likes a drop to drink, is going to find the adjustment very hard! Whereas a person who already enjoys eating healthily will find the anti-candida changes less arduous.

Supplements

Probiotics

Unlike antibiotics,probiotics replenish the families of friendly bugs living in the colon, and therefore they restore normal balance and displace candida.

There are various preparations on the market; the most effective are a mixture of Lactobacillus Acidophilus and Bifidobacteria. L. Acidophilus occurs in some yoghourt cultures, and can be bought in capsule, powder or tablet form. The most potent forms are marketed as Superdophilus, Vitaldophilus and Probion. Probion seems to be the most effective. (See Appendix A for suppliers.)

Probiotic supplements should be taken between meals, one capsule or 1/4 teaspoon of powder (or as instructed) three times a day. The L. Acidophilus and Bifidobacteria should multiply in the large bowel and gradually build up numbers to help the total amount of friendly bacteria, whose total weight may be between 3 and 5 lb.

Another way to take probiotics is to start your own yoghourt culture, using some of the organisms from the marketed probiotic preparations. This produces yoghourt with a more powerful brand of the correct bugs than most yoghourts bought over the counter. Some 'purists' have warned that milk and yoghourt should be avoided as the candida would be nourished by the milk. But the patient also needs this nourishment, especially the calcium and protein; so I would advise trying the yoghourt. If you find it upsets you then leave it out. Even people who are lactose intolerant can usually cope with yoghourt, because the lactobacilli and other bugs eat the lactose while they are turning the milk into yoghourt.

Supplements to help fight candida

Those suggested in Chapter 8 are ideal. The main ones recommended are:

- Vitamin C – 1 to 3 gms daily
- A good quality multi-vitamin and mineral (yeast free) preparation daily, giving vitamin A at least 7,000 units and vitamin B_6 at least 20 mg
- Zinc – 20–50 mg at night
- * Magnesium – 300–500 mg daily
- Calcium pantothenate 500 mg daily (especially if very allergic)
- Selenium – 100 IU daily
- Evening primrose oil, or Maxepa, at least 1,000 mg daily
- Vitamin E – 100–300 IU daily.

Note: * Magnesium seems to be especially important for people with candida infection. For some reason it does not appear to be absorbed, or else is lost to the system. Whatever the reason, at least 300 mg daily should be aimed at, and make sure you are getting vitamin B_6 in your daily pills.

Also especially helpful against candida are:

- Biotin 300 micrograms taken with acidophilus
- Garlic – either fresh as much as you can stand, in salads, etc., or garlic perles four to six daily
- Cold pressed olive oil about a tablespoon daily, such as on salads. It is the oleic acid which has natural anti-fungal properties. Perhaps this is why a lot of ME and candida symptoms seem to improve during a holiday to Greece or Spain.

Specific Anti-Fungal Medication

Nystatin and Amphotericin B (Fungilin)

These are the most commonly used agents to kill candida. There is little point in having treatment with nystatin without employing dietary means, because if the conditions in which candida flourished are not altered, then the symptoms will just keep on recurring. This is borne out by thousands of women with recurrent thrush, who have many repeated prescriptions of nystatin or other pessaries, but no advice about changing the body environment to discourage candida – so, naturally, all the nystatin does is to suppress the problem temporarily.

Nystatin comes in tablets, suspension (for babies and children), vaginal pessaries, and powder. For treating general symptoms of candida overgrowth, the powder preparation seems to work better than tablets.

Because the start of treatment frequently brings on more severe symptoms due to a 'die-off' reaction from dead and burst yeast cells, it is *essential to start with small doses*.

It is also best to start conquering the candida by starving it of sugar, so have at least two weeks on an anti-candida regime, plus probiotics and supplements before starting on nystatin or fungilin.

Dosage: Start with one tablet or 1/8 teaspoon a day. Each of these has 500,000 units of nystatin. After two days, increase to twice daily, and after another two days to four times daily – i.e. a total of four tablets or 1/2 teaspoon per day.

The powder does not dissolve well in water, but a good way to mix it is to put the day's total dose in a small bottle, such as an empty vitamin container, add water, and shake vigorously with the top screwed on. This mixture is taken, divided up into two or more lots, mixed with more water. This saves further mixing and stirring and you know you have taken the day's quota.

After two or three days, you may feel much worse. All the worst symptoms may be magnified, and you may feel quite awful – abdominal pains, sweating, headache, rapid pulse, insomnia, crying, etc. **Do not give up!** These signs mean that candida yeast spores are burst ing and dying, and releasing their toxins into the system.

Drink lots of water, take extra vitamin C and soldier on with the nystatin. After a further few days it will all get much better. If the reaction is really unbearable, carry on with nystatin but in a tiny dose for a few days, then start gradually building up again. There is no way of totally bypassing this reaction to the dying candida, so if you plan to start nystatin, do it at a time when you do not have important plans, or are on holiday; I realize that with ME important commitments were probably abandoned long ago, but you know what I mean.

Nystatin has a particularly bitter taste. If you cannot bear it, a little diluted fresh fruit juice such as apple (no added sugar of course) in the mixture is permissible.

The maximum dose of nystatin tolerated may be up

to 4 million units daily, i.e. eight tablets of 1/2 million each, or 1 teaspoon (heaped) of powder.

Powder or tablets? Tablets are much easier to take, avoid the taste, and are more easily obtainable on prescription in the UK.

However, powder reaches parts that tablets don't; candida lurks in the mouth, in gums, between teeth, in the throat, nose and gullet. If you can obtain powder *and* tablets, then a good compromise is to take powder when at home and tablets if you go out or away. When you take powder mixed up with water, keep the first mouthful in the mouth and swill it round for a few seconds before swallowing. This will get the nystatin into the cracks and crevices. You can gargle with it as well, especially if you have a sore throat, which may be due to candida as well as a virus.

Fungilin

This comes as lozenges, which are good to suck or chew to clear the fungus from the mouth and throat, but their dosage is too low to be effective in the gut.

As 100 mg tablets, fungilin is taken in a dose of one or two tablets four times a day. Similar 'die-off' symptoms may occur as with nystatin, and mean the treatment needs to be continued.

There does not seem to be any hard evidence on whether nystatin or fungilin works best. Which you have will probably depend on what is available on prescription in your country, and on your doctor's preference. Both are well tolerated, are not absorbed from the gut, and are effective against candida. One criticism of fungilin might be that it kills a broader range of yeasts than does nystatin, so could be accused of being too 'broad spectrum'. I am not sure that it matters, and different people will find one works better for them than the other.

Probiotics should be continued at the same time as taking nystatin or fungilin, which only destroy yeasts.

It may be necessary to treat candida in various other situations with different methods. Nystatin and fungilin can be used as lozenges, to treat mouth, throat and gullet; pessaries to treat vaginal infections; and creams for skin.

If large doses by mouth are not clearing the mental and gut symptoms, it may be worth administering nystatin direct to the lower bowel via an enema or even using pessaries as suppositories. This is best done by clearing the lower bowel with an ordinary enema, then giving a small retention enema of warm water containing 1/4 teaspoon of nystatin powder, or a crushed tablet of fungilin or nystatin. This is not an easy task for someone who is ill and weak, so unless a nurse or a helper who is trained to give enemas is at hand, this idea may not be practicable.

Treatment of candida may have to be continued for a year or more, and according to progress, the nystatin or fungilin can be cut down or stopped, and then the diet can be relaxed. However, vigilance needs to be maintained. If you get better and go on a binge of sugar, alcohol and cakes, you may get the candida back! In fact, once having kept off sweet things for months or years, few people want to regain a sweet tooth.

Colon cleansing by fibre

Some therapists advise adding special fibres such as oat bran fibre or psyllium husks to a diet high in vegetables. This helps remove old sticky putrefying matter from the lining of the colon. But you must drink a lot of water if you take psyllium husks, or there is a small risk of intestinal obstruction. A preparation of linseeds, e.g. Linusit, is safer than psyllium, and is recommended.

Colon cleansing by washouts

Colonic irrigation has apparently benefited some people with ME, and also some candida patients. At the present time, this therapy has not been subjected to any clinical trials, so any evidence for its usefulness is based on reports from some sufferers. The object of colonic irrigation is to remove sticky debris from the lining of the large bowel; this cleaning discourages build up of candida and other harmful bugs, and prevents toxic fermentation of waste matter. At the end of a cleaning session, during which water is introduced into the colon under controlled pressure, and flows out again, a preparation of acidophilus is left in the bowel.

As this procedure is not without potential hazards, *consult a properly trained colonic therapist* if you are considering this treatment. Some reports indicate that a large number of colon treatments may be needed to produce a good long-term effect, and the financial cost may be quite prohibitive. Colonic washouts are definitely *not* recommended for ME sufferers who are very unwell, and not as a first line treatment for probable candida overgrowth. There is usually a worsening of ME symptoms after the first few treatments, and in theory it is likely that viruses persisting in the gut may be 'stirred up' by the therapy and enter the blood stream.

There is a small risk of damage to the colon if the treatment is not done carefully; also there is loss of salts over a period with treatments done too close together, with resulting increase in muscle weakness.

Other Anti-Candida Treatments

Capristatin

Some fatty acids have been shown to destroy fungi; one such is caprylic acid, which is derived from coconuts. It is effective if taken as a slow release preparation, called capristatin, which reaches the large bowel before it is absorbed.

Capristatin may be very useful for anyone who cannot tolerate nystatin or fungilin. It is not obtainable on prescription.

Homeopathic Candida

Homeopathic practitioners may prescribe a potentized candida preparation, usually Candida 30x. This works on the usual homeopathic principle of 'treating like with like' (see Chapter 17). The patient should prepare for this by taking the anti-candida diet, supplements and probiotics for at least four weeks first. As with most homeopathic remedies, the candida nosode (as it is called) usually stirs up a reaction at the start of treatment, with worsening of most symptoms. As with taking nystatin or fungilin, this is a good sign albeit unpleasant, as it means the diagnosis of a candida problem was correct and that some improvement can be expected after the bad reaction has settled.

Anti-fungal foods

As previously mentioned, garlic, onion and vegetables of the cabbage family (brassicas) all have anti-fungal activity due to sulphur containing chemicals in them. They should all be eaten liberally, as well as olive oil for its oleic acid content.

Herbs

A tea made from a tree bark (taheebo tree) is reputed to have anti-fungal and immune system enhancing effects.

Aloe vera is a plant with anti-fungal properties. It is available in cream, ointment or lotion for external use, and also as a preparation to drink.

If you decide to have a go at getting rid of candida, you should first change your diet, then take some supplements and probiotics, and after a month or so consider having long-term anti-candida therapy.

If you have definite improvement in symptoms, then do keep on with the programme for at least six months. If there is absolutely no improvement in symptoms after three months on a diet and two months on anti-fungals, then you can say you have given it a fair trial and leave it. Many people who maintain that treating candida did not help them have not done the programme seriously and consistently.

Case History

The following story is typical of someone with ME and candida.

MRS C. A. AGED 42 (22 AT ONSET) HOUSEWIFE

She started her illness with a bad attack of flu at age of 20, then had two bad bouts of gastro-enteritis. At the time, she suffered from a bad marriage, overwork, damp house, and shortly before had had a lump removed from the breast. Blood and stool tests showed nothing.

After the illness started in 1968, with a bad dose of flu, I had constant diarrhoea and bad throats. My joints went haywire at the same time, the neck first, I had dreadful pins and needles in hands and feet. My jaw ached, it hurt to eat. I had severe abdominal pain and wind. I was very tired and lay on the floor by the fire when I could. My personality changed, with short temper and irritability. I felt awful most of the time. In 1969 we moved, I got tonsillitis again and again. Because of family trouble I saw a psychiatrist. *All the antibiotics I had gave me fungus in the mouth, I was given nystatin to suck.*

I remember craving sweet things, perspired a lot, got trembly if I didn't eat, and would drink 2 litres of coke a day.

In 1972 we moved again. I worked full time, still felt awful. Had more trouble with my neck, and trouble with the jaw. I started seeing a chiropractor.

My knees suddenly went, with dreadful pains. The hospital said it was probably 'arthritis caused by a virus'. I also had eczema (from 1969). I became allergic to many things – *all* painkillers brought me out in big lumps and I'd have difficulty breathing. Red wine made me short of breath, but not until 1985 did I find out all the foods I was allergic to.

I was given cortisone creams for my hands and face. My nerves were fragile, I tried tranquillizers and sleeping pills, but found them no good.

I am now getting better, but my symptoms were: Dreadful fatigue, any exercise made me feel drunk, or I had migraine or couldn't walk straight (felt drunk) the next day. Joint pains, muscle pains, PMT, blurred vision, feeling very cold, sweating, tinnitus, wind, bloating and diarrhoea, nerve pains, chest pains, difficulty breathing, and allergies. At present, improved, I can walk slowly for 1/2 hour on the flat, but feel whacked afterwards. If I rest before I have exhausted myself, I feel better and can avoid the headaches.

I started to feel better five or six years ago. I had remarried to a good man and felt content. *Then I tried to make myself fit* – jogging, aerobics, tennis, squash, I pushed myself, then started to go downhill. I also started a full-time degree course. After a year, throat problems came back, then a chest infection, and after that back came the tiredness, joint pains, blurred vision, etc.

I am now seeing a doctor at an allergy clinic. I am on a strict diet regime of vegetables, eggs, fish, meat, herb tea, garlic, onions, oils, psyllium husks. I eat no fruit yet, also no dairy products. I take acidophilus and vitamins. Acupuncture and homeopathy did not help.

I have had no sore throat for months, the eczema has gone, there is general improvement. I rest as well.

Past history

As a child I had blood poisoning several times from insect bites or little cuts.

By age 19, I had had four pregnancies, inflammation of the womb after the second (first two were miscarriages). I had wind and bloating of stomach from then on.

I had athlete's foot all through childhood, lots of mouth ulcers, and a fungus disease of the skin aged 16, and fungus infection in stitches after the first birth.

I used to eat yeast with sugar as a snack, also eggs

whipped up with sugar. I liked blue cheeses, pickles, and lots of coke – my diet was very poor.

[Comment – all the signs of fungus infestation right from her teens, yet no doctor spotted it. This story shows that ME and candida symptoms overlap. In her case, chronic yeast infection became much worse aged 20 following the virus infection. Is her diagnosis ME, or chronic candida?

She had a poor natural resistance to infection from childhood, the 'stage was set' to develop ME syndrome. Multiple allergies are frequently present with a yeast infection. Let us hope Mrs C. A. continues to get better on the anti-candida regime, and makes up for 20 years of ill health.]

Suggested Further Reading

The Yeast Connection, by William G. Crook (Professional Books, 1986).

Candida Albicans, by Leon Chaitow (Thorsons, 1985).

10
Allergies

The word *'allergy'* comes from two Greek words, *allos* meaning other, *ergon* meaning energy.

An allergy is an *altered reaction* to some outside stimulus. Something that provokes such an altered reaction is called an *allergen*.

Another word for an allergic reaction could be hypersensitivity. An allergic response is one that is different from the response of the majority of people; if you spill battery acid on your hands, you will get a nasty skin reaction; this is not an allergy, it is an acid burn, and is a normal reaction. Most people can breathe in grass pollens, a minority have hay fever. Most people can happily eat oranges, a small minority react to them.

The allergies that are easily recognized are: hay fever, asthma, eczema, migraine, skin reactions like nettle rash, and collapse after bee stings.

Hypersensitive reactions also occur to inhaled chemicals, to traces of chemicals in food and water, or even to apparently harmless common foods. The understanding of different types of allergy has broadened considerably in the last forty years, the pioneers of observation and research of food and chemical allergies being Dr Albert Rowe in the 1920s, and Dr Theron G. Randolph and colleagues in the USA in the 1950s.

A physician in the USA who specializes in treating allergics reckons that over 95 per cent of ME patients have allergies. Why is allergy so common a part of ME?

One explanation is that the immune system's defences initially act against infection, but do not switch off, because the virus becomes persistent. Instead, the immune system goes astray and becomes overactive to all the other foreign substances that enter the body. Certainly most ME people do have 'altered reactions' or allergy to many things which do not trouble healthy people.

Not everyone who has multiple allergies has ME, but, as with candida, there is considerable overlap between the conditions.

Allergies are of three types:

- *Ingested* – foods, liquids, chemicals in food
- *Inhaled* – pollen, house dust, house dust mite, moulds, animal fur; chemicals – formaldehyde, petrol, alcohol, aerosols, smoke and fumes.
- *Contact* – metals, e.g. nickel in bra and suspenders, rings, watches; dyes, various chemicals.

Having allergies is not a disease in itself, but is a symptom of an immune system which is not working properly. Therefore the successful management of allergies is not only to remove the allergens, but to help the immune system to recover. Of course, removing the stresses to the immune system, including exposure to allergens, is part of the treatment. The practical problems arise when a patient is found to be reacting badly to so many things that avoidance of them all means virtual starvation, lack of essential nutrients, and further stress from trying to avoid everything which causes a reaction.

For this reason, very restricted diets in ME may do more harm than good, except possibly for a short time to help diagnose food allergies. I have met people who are emaciated, weak and ill, who were trying to live on a very limited number of foods, having been given a list of twenty or more items to which they were apparently allergic on some sort of testing. These poor people had not been given any advice on supplements or how to correct the underlying problem, but had semi-starved for months and had become much worse. One big problem with a very limited diet is that one can become allergic to the few foods that one is eating.

Symptoms

Many ME symptoms are the same as those resulting from allergic reactions. Symptoms suggestive of allergies are:

- Symptoms worse *after* food, such as rapid pulse, wheezing, abdominal pains, bloating, sudden feeling of cold, headache, joint pain, sudden mood change, sweating;
- Symptoms improve on fasting;
- Great variations of symptoms through the day (this is typical of ME anyway);
- Feeling worse when in traffic jams, in city centres, on exposure to aerosol spray, fresh paint, etc., suggests chemical allergies;
- 'Better for being outside in fresh air' may not be just due to the daylight and sun, but may be because there are chemicals inside the building which are causing symptoms;
- Hay fever symptoms of sneezing and itchy eyes;
- Symptoms improving on change of location.

Allergic symptoms are so numerous, and include nearly all ME symptoms, that there is no point in making a list of them. It is the variability of them on exposure to different foods and chemicals that is typical of allergy.

If you suspect that food allergies, or intolerances as some doctors prefer to call them, are causing some of your problems, then adding details of what you eat and drink to your diary, or keeping a separate food diary, can be very helpful to pin-point culprit foods.

However, there may be foods which you eat every day that are making you ill. Instead of an acute reaction to something eaten rarely, such as swelling up and itching after strawberries, you can be chronically unwell by eating something so frequently that it never gets cleared from the system. This is called '*masked allergy*', and is also a form of addiction.

What happens is that constant exposure to the food leads to general ill health due to the constant stress on the immune system. (See also stress adaptation on page 184.) Avoidance of the allergen for twenty-four hours or more may lead to withdrawal symptoms, as happens when an alcoholic dries out, or a cigarette smoker stops smoking. These withdrawal symptoms settle down in a few days, then the subject becomes extra sensitive to the allergen and re-exposure causes much more dramatic symptoms than when it was being taken every day, when the allergic symptoms were masked through partial adaptation (or addiction really) to the substance.

The elimination and provocation-testing method of food allergy detection is based on understanding of this masked allergy phenomenon. If you avoid the suspect allergen, allow it to disappear from your gut, which takes up to five days, and then eat it again, it will cause the symptoms to reappear more strongly. If there is no ill effect, then it is regarded as safe.

The same principle applies to chemical masked

allergy. For example, a woman with chronic headaches, depression and fatigue went on holiday to a small Mediterranean island and after three days she felt wonderful. On returning home to a kitchen with a gas cooker, she felt absolutely dreadful, the depression and headache returned with a vengeance within a few hours of entering the house. Fortunately, the departure to a place of clean air had also sharpened the senses, and on entering the kitchen she detected a slight smell of gas, and later realized that was the culprit. Before going away, the chronicity of the symptoms masked the fact that it was a sensitivity to gas.

The mechanism by which one has symptoms from exposure to allergens is complex. Frequently it is not only one allergen but a combination of them plus other stresses which produces symptoms.

A good model for understanding is a barrel of water. If the level of water is too high it overflows. If the level of the sum total of stresses to one's body is too high, one has symptoms.

Another analogy is a ship afloat. She is laden down with all sorts of cargo, but so long as she stays afloat the ship is viable and can move. Add just a little more cargo and some high winds and waves and she will sink.

The final drop of water into the barrel and the final load of cargo are like the last straw that broke the camel's back. It is the sum total of all stresses that causes symptoms. So, then, if one can lower the level of water in the barrel, a further dollop of water may be all right and not cause symptoms. If the ship is not overloaded with cargo, a storm can come along and she will be safe.

Therefore any allergic patient may improve somewhat if he or she can jettison some cargo, to lower the sum total of stresses on the immune system. Very often the last straw is not a food allergy but is emotional or psychological stress. For example, a child with eczema very possibly has a cow's milk intolerance, masked because it is drunk daily; the child dutifully drinks the milk and is chronically miserable, itching or wheezing. When he or she goes to a new school, or has a row in the classroom, the eczema flares up very badly. Is the mental stress to blame, or the cow's milk? The answer is both, of course. But if the cow's milk is removed, probably the school stress will have less effect on the eczema.

In order to avoid contact with every possible allergen, one would need to live in an air-conditioned bubble, drink distilled water and starve. It is quite unrealistic for ME sufferers to try and avoid every single thing they react to, and there is some cause for concern if someone, who is already ill, semi-starves on a very strict elimination diet. So a lot of the management of allergies may have to be compromise.

Let us look at the various stresses and allergens that may be filling up your water barrel:

- Physical exercise
- Mental stress
- Airborne allergens – house dust, dust mite, pet hairs, pollens, etc.
- Electro-magnetic stress – TV, VDUs, power lines, etc.
- Chemical allergies – traffic fumes, aerosols, drinking water, gas leak, fresh paint, perfumes, new carpets, printing ink, etc.
- Minor food allergies – e.g. tomato, apple, pork
- Major food allergies – e.g. wheat, milk, sugar, coffee
- Virus infection.

Some of these things you cannot do anything about. It may be possible to move house if you live in a very polluted environment, but this is not feasible for everyone. What you should do is remove those things that you *can* do something about.

Detecting Food and Chemical Allergies

There are various ways of detecting food allergies.

Elimination, unmasking and challenge diet

This is the simplest and probably most accurate method of diagnosing food allergy. The disadvantage is that it is time consuming. *It should not be undertaken without medical supervision in any child, or a patient with depression, epilepsy or asthma,* because of the possibly dangerous consequence of a severe reaction on food testing after avoidance.

The patient either fasts for five days, drinking only spring water, or eats a few foods which are usually safe and which the patient rarely or never eats. Two foods are usually used, one fish or meat and one fruit, for example lamb, cod, pears, or some exotic fruit. During the fast, any symptoms are monitored and cravings for any particular foods are noted. If it is not a complete fast, it should be continued for at least a week to allow symptoms to clear up. If the patient still has all the original symptoms of the pre-fast period, then food allergy was probably not a factor, or else one of the foods used in the elimination period is not safe.

Following the fast, foods are reintroduced one at a time, each day, the less commonly eaten foods first. If there is a reaction on testing, it usually happens within 24 hours but may be delayed for 48 hours. All symptoms are noted, including the resting pulse rate before and up to two hours after a test food. A food which produces no reaction can be regarded as safe, and as testing proceeds the patient hopefully develops a gradually wider range of safe foodstuffs.

However, this method requires strong motivation and meticulousness on the part of the patient. Sometimes a delayed reaction may confuse the picture, and some foods, which if eaten together would cause symptoms, seem to be safe if tested separately.

Stone Age Diet

A modification of the Elimination Fast is the *Stone Age Diet*, taken for two weeks or more, followed by careful individual testing of things that have been left out.

The Stone Age Diet was first used in Britain for allergy testing and treatment by Dr Richard Mackarness, a psychiatrist at Basingstoke. The Stone Age Diet is arrived at by looking at the food our ancestors ate when man was still nomadic, before he became a farmer and grew crops intensively. The introduction of cereal crops, milk and milk products, sugar, tea, coffee and finally pollution of foods by agrochemicals and food additives, are all very recent changes in our diet. Obviously our metabolism and digestion has adapted to these changes with time, but logically the foods which are most likely to give trouble if one's adaptation breaks down are the more recently introduced ones.

Our ancestors, when hunter-gatherers, ate a wide range of raw plants – berries, roots, leaves, nuts, fruits. They would also catch and eat animal food – fish, shellfish, molluscs, small birds, rodents; as the hunting skills increased, larger game was eaten. The main diet was vegetarian, though, and provided high levels of vitamin C, and all minerals and vitamins; plus a lot of roughage, very little animal fat, and relatively more protein than in our modern diet. Wild animals, unlike intensively reared animals, had very little saturated fats, and certainly no chemical residues. In those early days, survival of the fittest was the rule; those humans who could not forage or hunt successfully did not survive, nor did any whose metabolism could not use the foods available to survive.

Because he ate a wide variety of things, according to the seasons, hunter–gatherer man did not tend to eat the same few things day after day throughout the year, so if allergies existed, they would not become masked. One assumes that if he ate sea slugs a few times and they made him ill, he did not try them again!

So the modern version of the Stone Age Diet aims to cut out the things *most likely* to be allergens, although our ancestors certainly did not eat exactly like this.

Stone Age Diet

Allowed	*Not allowed*
All meats and fish (fresh or frozen)	Grains (wheat, oats, rye, corn, rice, barley)
Fruit	Sugar – all kinds
Vegetables (fresh)	Milk and milk products
Potatoes	Eggs
Fresh nuts	Tea, coffee, alcohol
Pulses	Tinned, cured, or processed meat or fish
Spring water (glass bottled)	Anything tinned or processed
Pure vegetable oil	Dried fruit
	Tap water

This system works well if you are not allergic to any of the foods on the 'allowed' list. It is quite possible to eat the Stone Age Diet for months or years, and have complete nutrition and enough variety.

The main things to test, if two weeks or longer on the Stone Age Diet have improved your symptoms, are eggs, milk and its products, tap water and some grains. A good grain to test early is rice; it is less likely to cause symptoms than wheat or rye.

Eggs are important to test early as they are an excellent food, and it is socially difficult to avoid all grains completely. The sugar, tea, coffee, alcohol and processed foods you can do without, they are quite unimportant nutritionally.

If tap water causes a reaction, after testing on its own, then consider getting a water filter which removes chlorine, lead, aluminium and nitrates. There are cheap ones which need a filter cartridge changed every month, and expensive ones which are plumbed into the main tap. Bottled spring water can be used on outings, but is expensive to use all the time. People living in rural areas with clean air can collect rain-water, but it still needs to be filtered.

Of the grains, wheat (in UK) and corn (in the USA) are most likely to cause problems. You may be sensitive to the gluten, which is protein, or intolerant of the husk or bran. Some people with wheat intolerance can manage one slice of unprocessed white bread a day or twice a week, but get symptoms if they go back to four slices of wholemeal bread a day. Oats have less gluten, and if tolerated are a better source of fibre than wheat. Rice is rarely allergenic, perhaps because it is not part of our staple diet, and is low in gluten. Unrefined rice is a good substitute as a starch for wheat.

Other methods of allergy detection depend on various tests, and different ones are used by different doctors.

Cytotoxic testing

A sample of your blood is taken, and the white blood cells are separated out. The white cells are exposed to a range of foods and chemicals, and their reaction is examined using a microscope. The reactions are graded from no reaction, a mild reaction (the cells change shape) to a severe reaction (the cells die). The correlation between the results of the test and improvement following avoidance is fairly good, but the test is expensive and can only be performed at a few specialized centres. It tends to give a long list of allergens; however in practice one avoids only the items which have given a severe or moderate reaction. One advantage is that chemicals can be tested for, whereas an elimination diet only sorts out foods.

Intradermal testing and neutralization technique

This procedure is used by several clinical ecologists. It is expensive and time consuming, and patients can have reactions which last for hours and confuse subsequent tests.

A minute dose of a solution of test substance in saline is injected into the skin to raise a small bleb. The diameter of the bleb is measured, and after exactly two minutes the bleb is examined again. If it has increased in size, particularly if there is redness of the surrounding skin, or symptoms in the patient, this indicates a positive reaction. Successive diluted doses of the test substances are injected and measured, until a dilution is reached which causes no reaction. This strength commonly 'switches off' any general symptoms and reduces the reaction in previous blebs. It is recorded as the neutralizing dilution, or 'end point'.

The patient is given drops or injections containing the neutralizing strengths of the major antigens, to use to protect against allergic reactions. This can be very useful for a multiple allergic subject, who can then eat some offending foods with this protection. It is also very valuable for severely chemically allergic people, who react to minute amounts of chemicals which cannot be avoided in their environment.

The disadvantage is the time needed to test for everything (one may spend a whole morning reaching the end point of one test substance!), and the fact that in a highly allergic person the end points can and do change, and the desensitizing drops may have to be worked out over and over again.

The mechanism by which this neutralization and desensitization works is not fully understood, but is probably electrical. In high dilutions, there may be no original molecules left of the allergen, as in homeopathic remedies.

Applied Kinesiology, or the muscle weakness test

In this test, which requires no sophisticated equipment, the test substance itself or a vial containing a solution of it, is placed in contact with the patient, usually over the centre of the body at the umbilicus. The patient is lying relaxed, and first the strength of action of one or more arm muscles is assessed, then retested after the test substance has been placed in contact. It is not a trial of strength, and very small movements are tested. If the patient reacts to the item being tested, there is an immediate perceptible weakness of the muscle.

Some testers use successive dilutions of test substances until the dilution at which normal muscle strength returns is reached. This end point can be used to make neutralizing drops as described in the intradermal test.

This method, often called AK, is fairly accurate with a skilled tester, but not everyone can develop this skill. It has the advantage of being non-invasive, quick, and does not produce unpleasant symptoms. With a skilled practitioner, the test has almost 100 per cent reproducibility if a patient is tested on consecutive days. Ideally the patient does not know what substance is being tested at each test.

The Vega test

The mechanism of this test is electrical, as must be the Applied Kinesiology test. The patient holds an electrode which is connected to an instrument that measures electrical resistance. A probe is placed over an acupuncture point and this completes a circuit. A reading is taken on the Vega machine, and then a test substance is introduced into the circuit, and the electrical reading changes if this substance has had some effect on the resistance.

The test is quick and without side effects, but, as with AK, requires skill on the part of the tester.

None of these methods is 100 per cent accurate, and in a very sensitive person the allergies can change from day to day. However, the most important sensitivities come up repeatedly on subsequent testing; these are the ones that the patient needs to avoid.

Treatment of Food and Chemical Allergies

(1) Avoidance of allergens where possible.
(2) Correction of any nutrient deficiencies, and supplements to strengthen the immune system.
(3) Desensitization by neutralizing drops or injections.
(4) Enzyme Potentiated Desensitization.
(5) Oral sodium cromoglycate – Nalcrom.

Avoidance

For the majority of allergic people, avoidance of a few main foods, and cleaning up the chemical environment as far as possible, combined with nutritional measures, is the best way. If a major food allergen, such as wheat, is avoided for six months or so, the patient may become less sensitive and may be able to tolerate it eaten in small amounts once or twice a week. If it is eaten daily and in increasing amounts, then a masked allergy may develop again. Some allergies are 'fixed' for life, and a long spell of avoidance does not change the sensitivity. There is often some enzyme deficiency associated with these allergies. Most patients find out if they have a lifelong allergy to something such as strawberries or shellfish, which are not eaten daily.

However so called *milk allergy* is commonly due to deficiency of *lactase*, the enzyme needed to digest lactose. This is usually lifelong, is very common in Asians and Africans and occurs in about 30 per cent of Europeans. Lactose intolerance sometimes develops following some gastro-intestinal infection, such as a bug called Giardia Lamblia (commonly picked up overseas), and also enteroviruses (such as in ME). Some milk sensitive people can tolerate milk if it has been treated with a lactose reducing enzyme. Other milk sensitivities may be reacting to the cow's milk protein, yet tolerating goat's or sheep's milk. If you are allergic to cow's milk, it is worth asking for separate tests for milk protein and lactose.

Often avoidance of one or two chief food allergens will reduce the overall load and allow you to eat other things to which you are less sensitive. If the less sensitive foods are eaten no more than once every four days, or perhaps twice a week, there is less chance of masked allergy developing. This is the principle behind the *Rotation Diet*, which can be used both for managing and diagnosing allergies.

The Rotation Diet means you have different foods each day and allow four days before eating something again. Because of cross sensitivity, a strict rotation diet includes members of the same food family in the four-day rule – e.g. neither chicken nor eggs must be eaten again before four days. A rotation diet can be interesting to create on paper, using columns for food groups for each day. In practice it can be quite tedious to stick to, and you cannot use up leftovers the next day. It can be quite unworkable if you have to cater for the rest of the family, and makes eating out very awkward (as do most exclusion diets).

Enzyme Potentiated Desensitization

This technique was developed by Dr Len McEwen at St Mary's Hospital, London.

A mixture of minute doses of highly purified antigens is combined with an enzyme called Beta-glucuronidase, which potentiates the effects of the antigens, plus two other chemicals.

This solution is introduced in one of two ways. It can be injected into the skin, to raise a small bleb. Or else it is placed in contact with the skin on the patient's inner forearm in a small cup, the skin having been scratched beforehand to break the superficial layers. The solution of antigens and enzyme is left in contact with the skin for 24 hours, or less if a severe reaction develops.

A great number of antigens can be included in the mixture, maybe 70 or more, so it is not necessary to have established the patient's individual sensitivities.

EPD is repeated at monthly intervals for three to four months, but the benefits, i.e. increasing tolerance to foods, do not develop for six to 12 months after starting treatment. When it does work, the improvement seems to be permanent, unlike desensitizing drops or injections. EPD is expensive and the results are not instant, and in Britain it is only available at a few centres and not in the National Health Service. However those who complete the course report good results, which are more permanent than other methods of desensitization.

Nalcrom – sodium cromoglycate

This drug is better known by asthmatics, who inhale it from a puffer to prevent allergic asthma attacks. The drug works by blocking the reaction of certain cells (called mast cells) to the antigen and antibody, so that the chemical substances which cause the allergic effects – inflammation, wheezing, headaches, etc. – are not released. Mast cells exist scattered in the membranes lining nose, throat, lung airways and also the gut.

Nalcrom can be taken in capsules just before meals, and seems to be effective in preventing food allergy reactions in about two-thirds of patients who try it. It is not a substitute for sensible avoidance of main food offenders, but could be very useful to someone who is allergic to many main foods, and also in a situation where the allergic person copes well at home, but has problems travelling or visiting. It is only available on prescription, comes in 100 mg capsules, and dosage for an adult is 100 to 200 mg three times daily. It seems fairly safe; occasional side effects are nausea, joint pains or rashes.

Suggested Supplements for Allergic People

First, ensure that any supplements you obtain are free from gluten, sugar, yeast, grains and colourings.

The regime suggested for an ME sufferer on page 123 is quite suitable.

The main deficiencies which occur in very allergic people are of B vitamins, iron, zinc, magnesium and essential fatty acids.

Dealing with bowel bug overgrowths such as candida (see Chapter 9) may improve food intolerances quite dramatically.

Taking probiotics such as acidophilus and other preparations, to help re-establish normal balance of bowel organisms, is advisable (see page 137).

A Word of Caution about Food Allergies

If you have lost weight with ME, are already underweight, or have severe symptoms, do not undertake elimination diets without specialized medical supervision. By further reducing the nutritional intake, you may become worse. If possible, seek advice from a medically trained clinical ecologist, or an NHS allergist.

If you want to try and sort things out for yourself and have no medical help, a suggested routine is:

First – follow the diet guidelines outlined in Chapter 7, avoid all chemicals in food, and take the suggested nutritional supplements. This may improve symptoms after two months.

Second – if you suspect food allergies, either try the Stone Age Diet, and eat plenty of vegetables, meat, fish and fruit; or try cutting out completely either wheat or cow's milk, one at a time, as these are the commonest offenders.

Third – reduce other possible allergens as much as possible, i.e. chemicals around you.

Suggested Further Reading

Not All in the Mind, by Dr Richard Mackarness (Pan, 1976).
The Food Allergy Plan, by Keith Mumby (Allen & Unwin, 1985).
Allergies: Your Hidden Enemy, by Theron G. Randolph and Ralph W. Moss (Thorsons, 1980).

11

Chemical Sensitivity

This problem seems to be increasing. You only have to consider the vast array of products made from petrochemicals (hydrocarbons) which have become part of twentieth-century living, to see that we cannot possibly expect humans to have adapted to them in such a short time.

Rachel Carson's classic book, *Silent Spring*, written back in 1962, was a chilling forecast of the price we may have to pay for tampering with the environment. Talking about the effect of DDT and other pesticides on living creatures and food chains, she said in 1962, 'It looks as if we will go on swallowing these chemicals whether we like it or not and their real effect may not be seen for another twenty or thirty years.'

Most ME sufferers seem to have an increased degree of sensitivity to chemicals compared to when they were well, and chemical allergy goes with food allergy. Some reactions are obvious; for example someone who gets a headache and watering eyes when they open the morning newspaper is probably sensitive to the printer's ink or other chemicals in the paper. However, there may be other more insidious symptoms, harder to relate to the cause. Someone who is very sensitive may be unwell on days when the wind blows in a direction from some chemical factory 30 or 40 miles away. The presence of a smoker in the household may cause chronic worsening of symptoms in a susceptible non-smoker.

Short of moving to a remote place by the sea,

drinking spring water and growing your own food organically, you may feel that you have little control over your environment. You can support pressure groups such as Friends of the Earth, Greenpeace, and the Campaign for Lead Free Air, and write to your MP, Euro MP, and the appropriate Minister about environmental issues.

Nearer to home there is quite a lot you *can* do to clean up your immediate environment.

What are the Chemicals Most Likely to Cause Problems?

Hydrocarbons, or fossil fuels	*Where found*
Petrol, diesel, oils	Motor vehicles, boat engines
Paraffin (kerosene)	Lawnmowers, oil-fired boilers
Natural or calor gas	Gas central heating, gas stoves, gas cylinders, pipes
Coal, coke, anthracite	Smoke or fumes from coal fires or stoves
Wood, charcoal	Smoke from wood fires, stoves, barbecues

Hydrocarbon derivatives

People who are sensitive to petrol, gas, diesel and smoke are usually affected by most hydrocarbon products.

Plastics	Wrappings, bottles, clingfilm, plastic food boxes, furnishings

Synthetic textiles	E.g. nylon, terylene, dralon, in clothing, carpets and upholstery
Paints, varnish, solvents	Newly decorated houses and offices
Aerosol propellants	Hair spray, deodorants, fly spray, spray paint, air fresheners, cleaning agents, etc.

Detergents, polishes, cosmetics, perfumes, cleaning fluids (e.g. dry cleaners, carpet cleaners), sponge rubber, scented soaps, wax candles.

Phenol products

Carbolic acid – (this is pure phenol)
Dettol and other antiseptics
Many preservatives
Pesticides, herbicides
Polyurethane foam
Dyes
Bakelite and other hard plastics

Formaldehyde

If you feel unwell in a large clothing store, it is formaldehyde affecting you.

Dyes, fabric finishes, proofings, in textiles
Traffic fumes
Fertilizers
Insecticides
Foam rubber
Fabric conditioner
Paper manufacture, printing ink
Photography
Most building materials, cavity wall insulation; and formaldehyde occurs in many other things

Food colourings

The following foods usually have synthetic colourings:

Glace cherries
Coloured ice creams, sweets, lollipops
Most fruit 'squashes'
Yellow cheeses
Coloured cakes and icing
Many canned soft drinks
Many processed foods

The correct procedure is to check the label when buying foods. Most items listed above should be avoided by ME sufferers anyway.

Colourings in medicines

This source of potential trouble is easy to overlook. What is iniquitous is that many *children's* medicines are still coloured or flavoured with synthetic chemicals, many of which are banned in countries outside the UK.

Hopefully, ME sufferers reduce drug taking to the absolute minimum. If a medicine you really need is suspiciously coloured, your pharmacist should be able to inquire of the manufacturers what the contents are. Sometimes people who have a 'drug reaction', perhaps a skin rash or abdominal pains, may be allergic to some substance other than the medicine itself.

Chemicals in tobacco smoke

You do not need to be a smoker to be affected by the fumes from other people's smoke from cigarettes, pipes or cigars. The smoke contains many chemicals, and a sensitive person can be affected by traces lingering in a smoker's clothes or hair. If you or someone in your household or place of work smokes, then avoiding all the other sources of chemical pollution may be a waste of time. You are entitled to a smoke-free place at work these days, and you must make your home a smoke-free zone if you are serious about improving your health.

Steps You Can Take to Minimize Chemical Pollution

You and those around you must stop smoking!

On your person – wear natural fibres if possible. Avoid fabrics with special finishes. Avoid clothes that have to be dry cleaned, or else air them well after cleaning. Make sure your clothes are thoroughly rinsed, use soap powders or flakes, or ecologically safe detergents, and avoid fabric softeners in the wash.

If you shop for clothes, look for cottons,pure wools, etc., and if a garment has any odour, don't buy it, or wash it several times before wearing it.

Cotton/terylene mixes are better than pure nylon.

Do not use perfume, aftershaves, deodorants, scented soaps (coal tar soaps included) or talcum powder, synthetic fragrances and bubbles in the bath. Avoid hair sprays, setting gels, and hair creams, scented shampoos or conditioners.

Women should ideally stop using make-up, but using natural products, such as those found in the Body Shop and similar, may be of positive value psychologically.

The bathroom and bedroom are therefore potentially full of unnecessary chemicals which are applied to the body.

In the house – while in the bathroom, look for and remove air fresheners, toilet deodorizers, and cleaning agents. The bath and WC can be cleaned with the least smelly agents possible, and these can be kept in a cupboard somewhere else or outside. It is a myth, fostered by advertising agencies, that a smell of 'pine' or 'meadow freshness' equals hygiene. Women brought up during a less chemical era will remember that bathrooms could be kept clean without all these smells.

Look under the sink, and see what cleaning agents you can jettison. Those you decide to keep, such as washing up liquid and unperfumed sink cleaner perhaps, keep tightly sealed, and in the cupboard. Furniture polishes, 'instant clean' liquids for floors, sprays, etc., should all go out. There is little that cannot be cleaned with water, soap, or bicarbonate of soda. It is better to have a less shiny home with occupants less allergic, than a shiny home smelling of 'pine' or whatever and its occupants ill.

Paints, solvents, etc., should be stored outside in a shed or garage. Plans for redecorating should be postponed until either you are better, or you can go away while it is done and not return until the smell has cleared.

It is probably not practical to rip up all wall-to-wall foam-backed carpets, but if you are very allergic, it might be worth taking up such a carpet from your bedroom, and having the old linoleum which may be underneath, or bare floorboards with woollen rugs or carpets. The test of such carpets is if you can smell them when you come inside.

Very sensitive, ill people find benefit from creating one room in the house which is as chemical free as possible, a 'safe haven', with natural cotton curtains, no plastics, no treated furniture, no foam, and no treated wallpaper. Many modern wallpapers are treated with fungicides, and cause trouble for some time.

If you are replacing any furniture, try and avoid

foam-filled furnishings with synthetic, or imitation leather covers. Basically, anything *new* is likely to be chemically treated in some way. Safer replacement furnishings might be found in second-hand shops, but beware of woodworm treated wood. The best furnishings are of wood, or metal, with cotton or wool covers, kapok cushions, etc.

One problem area is the bed. Should you have feather-filled or foam-filled pillows? Good quality feather pillows are better if you are not allergic to them. A lot of allergic reactions to beds and bedding are due to the ubiquitous house-dust mite, which establishes itself in all soft furnishings. Covering the mattress and pillows with finely woven cotton 'ticking' helps. Washable wool or cotton blankets can be kept free of dust mites, and the best duvet would be feather filled but washable.

In the kitchen, see if you can use glass or china food containers instead of plastic in the fridge, and avoid plastic bags or clingfilm. Greaseproof paper is still around and is better for wrapping. Cooking utensils should be of stainless steel, Pyrex, cast-iron or enamelled ware.

Aluminium pans are bad for anyone, as aluminium is poisonous and small amounts enter cooking food, especially stewed fruit. Special non-stick linings to pans may be convenient, but the chemicals they contain can contaminate your food. In any case, when the non-stick surface is past its prime, then foods will stick and burn far worse than on an old cast-iron pan.

More difficult to get rid of in your home is a heating system which might be releasing minute quantities of fumes that are affecting you. Also it may not be easy to find out whether it is a culprit. Most people in the UK in urban areas seem to have North Sea gas heating – it is worth having the appliance thoroughly serviced regularly and tested for leaks. A gas cooker is relatively easy to replace by electric, and gas cookers are a common source of minute traces of gas, even from a pilot light. One way to test if gas is causing a problem is to go and stay somewhere with no gas at all and see if you improve. On returning, if you can smell any trace of gas at all, you are probably hypersensitive to it.

Alternatively, switch off the gas at the meter for two weeks, ventilate the house well, and then see if any symptoms return when it is switched on again. This test may not be so clear as going away, because traces of gas persist from pipes and connections.

Many ME sufferers seem to get worse from November to March. I wonder if being indoors most of the day with gas heating and other indoor chemicals is as much to blame as is lack of sunshine and daylight?

Indoor pollution is worse than outdoor pollution, unless you live beside a motorway junction or chemical works. At least outdoor pollution gets blown away sometimes by a good wind in the right direction. A lot of people never open any windows in the house. Fear of burglary and of losing heat may be the reasons. But even in winter, each room should be ventilated once a day for a while, especially on windy days when the outside air is cleaner.

Other sources of indoor pollution are 'dry rot' treatments, timber treatments, certain cavity wall insulations (foam), smokers, damp and moulds (adequate ventilation should prevent these), portable gas heaters, paraffin heaters, coal or oil-fired stoves, and houses that have been treated with insecticides, also air conditioning units and any other motorized machinery.

Televisions and VDU screens, when in operation, give off formaldehyde, because of their plastic components and casing. They also give off positive ions, gamma radiation, and electromagnetic fields, which are harmful to ME sufferers and indeed to everyone. This may be why so many ME people cannot tolerate much television.

One person commented that he had the same ill effects by sitting in front of a TV with his eyes blindfolded to avoid visual disturbance, as he had if he actually watched the programme. His symptoms were: spaced-out feeling, headache, increased mental 'fog' and blurred vision for up to 24 hours after exposure to TV.

On the whole, a radio is probably less harmful to the brain. A solution for users of VDU screens, for example those sufferers who use them at work or those who have bought a word processor to write a book at home, is to get a special screen which blocks off the harmful rays. A negative ionizer sat beside your screen and pouring negative ions into the air also helps.

A fairly drastic step is to move house. This may be considered if someone with ME has tried everything to clean up the amount of indoor chemicals, but is still very ill. Obviously there is no point in giving up a home with gas heating and moving to an idyllic country cottage surrounded by crop fields which are regularly sprayed! So if such a step is taken, it is important to look for somewhere with electric heating, or a boiler well away from the house, in a relatively unpolluted area away from busy roads.

With the banning of coal fires in many cities, the air may be cleaner than in some parts of the countryside as mentioned above, if you can find a quiet area with plenty of greenery. Old houses may be unsafe because of treatment for timber and dry rot. Probably the best homes ecologically are those built between 1920 and 1960.

Avoiding tap water has been discussed earlier. It is rather silly to replace all your saucepans and refrigerator boxes and then eat food full of chemicals. As mentioned in Chapter 7, organically produced food is best; the more that people ask for it, the more will become available.

What to do if you have an acute reaction to a chemical

Drink a glass of water containing one gram of vitamin C and a level teaspoon of bicarbonate of soda. Repeat the vitamin C at hourly intervals and continue to drink lots of fluids for 24 hours.

This helps neutralize the reaction, and gives a boost to the white cells and adrenals. Whatever the mechanism, this remedy *does* help, so keep vitamin C handy if you travel, and at hand in the home.

At home, change your clothes and have a shower, to remove traces of the allergen from clothes and skin.

Go outside (if inside), or open a window and breathe deeply of clean air. If in a car, shut all windows and vents, and try and get away from whatever it is – crop sprays, road works, or a queue of buses.

Desensitization

Desensitization to chemicals and foods can be carried out after testing by intradermal skin testing, applied kinesiology or Vega testing, and establishing neutralizing strengths. Some clinical ecologists treat very sensitive patients in a special ecologically safe unit, where everything is done to create a chemical free environment. Many sufferers improve dramatically while in these surroundings, and can return home with a supply of desensitizing drops or injections.

This is fine, so long as the patient also takes steps to clean up the home as much as possible and also tries to correct any nutritional deficiencies. But in many sufferers, chemical allergy symptoms return after a time unless the underlying abnormality of immune function is corrected.

Avoidance of all possible allergens will help the immune system, and so should be attempted by ME sufferers as part of the self-help plan.

Case History

The following story is of someone who found chemical avoidance helpful. It also illustrates that many health workers still do not understand the symptoms of ME.

MRS L. C. AGE 28 EX-HAIRDRESSER

Her illness started in 1982, suddenly. She has been ill since then – now six years.

> I believe long-term exposure to chemicals at work, i.e. hairsprays, perms, bleaches, etc., whittled away at my immune system over the years; then in the year previous to the onset I was working long hours. So when I went down with the infection it was severe, and I think my powers of recovery were not a quarter of what they should have been.
>
> My symptoms were, and are:
>
> Feeling very ill, muscle weakness and pain, strange sensations in the head,pain in all muscles especially thighs, excessive perspiration, gid-

> diness, cold feet and hands, tingling in lower gums, wheezing, palpitations, pain as though I had 'acid' coursing through my veins.

She had a muscle biopsy and blood tests done two years after the onset; the muscle biopsy was abnormal, and the diagnosis was myalgic encephalomyelitis. She had myocarditis three years ago. She has been virtually bedridden and permanently fatigued for most of five years. During the last year there has been some improvement.

> **Ridding my home of all chemicals** has produced a dramatic improvement. After being totally collapsed and bedridden for over a year an ME sufferer/patient of Dr Monro's told me to move house and clear out at least my bedroom of all allergens or I would be bedridden for the rest of my life! It made sense. My ex-home had been totally renovated and sprayed with fungicide (for dry rot) and pesticide (for woodworm). Also I lived in a top floor flat on a busy road which fed the pier and rail station, my carpets were foambacked, my furniture was chipboard and hardboard, I surrounded myself with perfumes and spent a fortune in the body shop so every bath had scented oils and bubble bath in. We were advised to buy a home which was 15 to 20 years old (older would likely have been sprayed and treated for dry rot, damp, etc.).
>
> We lifted the carpet in our new bedroom and luckily there were cream coloured hard vinyl tiles underneath which cleaned up well. We use all 100 per cent cotton sheets and night attire and got rid of our modern furniture (which gives off formaldehyde). I gave away all my perfume and now buy SIMPLE toiletries, also we use Boots washing up

liquid and automatic soap powder for sensitive people. I'm phasing out my clothes which are made of synthetic fabrics. I don't allow anyone to smoke in my house and I ask friends and family not to wear perfume, aftershave, or hairspray when visiting.

A friend was wearing hairspray when visiting recently, I didn't like to say anything at first. After one and a half hours I went from being able to sit quite easily to collapsed and unable to hold myself up – could hardly believe the effect it had on me! After she'd gone it took two hours for the air to clear with the door open – when it did clear and I had gulped in lots of fresh air I could *sit* once again. I would advise all bedridden or severely affected people to take the same advice, remembering *all family members* must switch to unscented toiletries.

I feel that the conventional medical profession is light years away from understanding even the most basic and fundamental truths about the nature of this illness.

In June of this year I had a dreadful experience. I was horrifically unwell and living with my parents as we had just sold our flat. My husband had just started his new job and was in agony with three slipped discs in his back. I was totally incapacitated and unable to wash myself or get to the toilet unaided.

In desperation I wrote to Dr W. at . . . hospital and they took me in. I was carried out on a stretcher as I couldn't sit or stand. The first day wasn't too bad, except the nurses wanted me to walk a very long corridor to the toilet – it was agony, I couldn't hold myself up.

I tried to explain that I couldn't sit up in bed for my meals, they wanted me to sit at a table. The staff could see how disabled I was because they had trundled me away in an ambulift for a bath, which I just slumped in, totally unable to move. On the third day they wanted me to go to the gym for physiotherapy, I tried again to explain how terribly ill I felt and couldn't even sit up. On the fourth day I was still under great pressure to go for physio. Again I tried to explain how ill I felt and how I felt sucked to the bed like an iron filing to a magnet.

It was the last straw when the nurse said to me at lunchtime, 'Do you *want* to sit at the table?' I just lost control, and screamed at her in floods of tears, and told everyone of them that I was not trying to be uncooperative, that I was not a lazy creature that enjoyed lying in bed. The sister tried to change my mind about signing myself out. I agreed to see Dr W. as I was grateful that he took me in at short notice, but he called me selfish, and said I had an abnormal attitude and that the reason I had been bedridden for over a year was because I had put down 'clamps' and was afraid of trying. I realized just how much the 'research hospital' knew about ME. Nothing.

I just want to forget it all now and concentrate on getting better which I feel quietly confident about. I believe our healing to a large extent comes from within ourselves and that self help should mean exactly that. I have kept a diary since I've been ill and have come to a number of conclusions about this illness which I am trying to get down on paper hoping to help others.

Things which have helped

- Relaxation tapes.
- Home help – had over 25 phone calls in response to advert.

- Personal stereo (ideal for listening to relaxation tapes, etc., when bedridden).
- Massage – various books available.
- Meditation.
- Hot bath – helps inflammation and vein pain (not too hot).
- Fresh air – as much as possible.
- Christian counselling – ask at your local Christian bookshop for this service. Good for Christians and non-Christians.
- Christian healing – local church prayer groups usually have a healing ministry.
- Chemical avoidance – read *Chemical Children*.

Suggested Further Reading

Chemical Victims by Dr Richard Mackarness (Pan, 1980).
Chemical Children: how to protect your family from harmful pollutants, by Peter Mansfield and Jean Monro (Century, 1987).

12

Stress, Meditation

What is Stress, and Why Does it Cause Illness?

The word 'stress' is quite fashionable nowadays, and is blamed for much ill health. But what do we mean by stress?

It is comfortable to think that stress is something which just happens to us, like a car accident or a dose of flu – or ME. Some stresses are like that, the unexpected car crash, the terrorist attack, floods and earthquakes. With this point of view we can allow ourselves to believe that we have no control over how much stress we receive. We can say: 'Life has treated me badly, that is why I have become ill.' This is the attitude of a 'victim'. Or we can say: 'There are so many demands made of me, I am exhausted', or 'I have to strive and strive at work, to keep my position in society' – these are attitudes of people who think they have stress put on them by situations beyond their control.

Just as germs do not themselves cause fever, but the body's reaction to germs causes symptoms of infection, so stress itself does not lead to ill health, it is how stress is handled which determines if we are adversely affected.

Stress means any change in our environment which tries to knock us off course, and to which there is a bodily reaction to put us back on course; or, anything which disturbs our equilibrium, our 'homeostasis', of mind or body.

'For every action there is a reaction'; this is one of Newton's laws of physics. The whole tendency of the living person is towards stability, whether stability of blood sugar, of temperature, or of emotional well-being. So 'stress' has a much broader definition than the stress of a demanding job or a demanding family. It can be climatic – changes of heat or cold, hunger, poisons, trauma, chemical pollution, any infection, exhaustion, lack of sleep, fear, anxiety.

Dr Hans Selye, Professor of Experimental Medicine and Surgery at the University of Montreal, has studied the effects of stress on living things since the 1930s. He was the first to show that the adrenal gland cortex produces cortisone in response to any disturbance to the body, and that cortisone is part of the defence reaction. Selye performed careful experiments on rats, using exposure to severe cold as the stress. He observed three stages in the animals' response to repeated exposure to cold:

(1) A shock response to the first exposure to the stress followed by the animals' reaction, and then recovery.
(2) On repeated exposure the animals appeared to adapt, and to become resistant to the cold. In this stage, the adrenal glands enlarged, and a stimulus from the pituitary gland (below the brain) to the adrenals via a hormone called ACTH increased. The changes in the animals to counteract the stress become more permanent.

    The rats appeared to be coping.
(3) Exhaustion. Selye observed that the rats gradually failed to thrive, and in those that died, a post mortem showed that the adrenal glands had given up their fight, and were shrunken and had ceased functioning.

Selye called these events the *general adaptation syndrome*.

These stages are similar in humans.

(1) The first exposure to stress produces an outpouring of cortisone, and also of adrenaline to prepare the body for 'fight or flight' – the initial arousal state. If the stress passes, this reaction settles, and the body returns to its status quo.
(2) Repeated stressing leads to a stage of adaptation. However the arousal changes become more or less permanent; the person may appear to adapt, but the general health declines and there are chronic symptoms such as migraine, asthma, rashes, blood pressure, heart problems, indigestion, palpitations, mental problems and unstable blood sugar control. The body cannot remain in a constant state of arousal by stress and constantly trying to restabilize, without permanent damage.
(3) In stage three there is a breakdown in the adaptation. The result is collapse and exhaustion. This may take the form of a heart attack, nervous breakdown, or perhaps a major illness such as cancer. The breakdown of the body's adaptation may occur following an apparently minor stress.

The second stage of the general adaptation syndrome is the one in which most GPs see their patients, with a whole range of chronic non-life-threatening illnesses. At this stage, if the stress is removed, whatever it is, recovery can take place.

In ME, the viral infection which appeared to trigger it off may have been the 'last straw' for a chronically stressed system, leading to literal exhaustion and collapse. I know that this point of view will upset some ME sufferers, who will angrily say, 'I was perfectly well with no stress before I went down with the infection which left me with ME, therefore my present illness must be entirely caused by the virus.'

The trouble is that the very idea that one has been under stress, has not handled it properly, and therefore become ill, implies a weakness of character or that getting ill was all one's own fault; this of course is very hard to bear for someone whose life is devastated by ME.

But maybe the chronic stress was not emotional, nor overwork. Perhaps it was exhaustion through bringing up small children. Perhaps it was a serious accident followed by months of convalescence, or maybe long-term exposure to chemicals and developing a masked allergy to them. There are lots of ways of being repeatedly stressed. What really matters, if you reach the stage of 'exhaustion' and become seriously ill, is to accept where you are, to stop struggling to adapt, and to try to reverse the situation of the exhausted adrenal glands.

Having ME is of course a continuing new stress and some people allow it to get them down more than others. Various ways of reducing the effects of stress are recommended. These might be meditation, relaxation, and learning to breathe properly; there is also counselling, which may help to give insight into the reality of becoming ill and the possibility of getting better.

Meditation

Meditation is an excellent way of obtaining rest for the mind and the body. There are several ideas about meditation which are untrue, and may discourage people from learning it.

Popular misconceptions about meditation

- Meditation is thought to require effort to control the mind, and thus to be difficult and mentally taxing.
- It is supposed to be appropriate only for a particular lifestyle – of recluses, mystics, religious people who withdraw from the world.
- It is associated with oriental religions such as Buddhism and Hinduism; and many people erroneously believe that you need to join a sect or convert to a different faith to practise meditation.
- Most people do not know about any of the benefits of meditation; they think it is done only to achieve a state of spiritual enlightenment.

However, since 1958, the practice of transcendental meditation has been rediscovered and made available to anyone throughout the world, by a system of teaching and learning which is handed on from person to person. This was the result of the work of Mahareshi Mahesh Yogi, an Indian scholar and teacher, who did not invent TM, but rather revived it and also instituted scientific research into its effects and benefits.

Facts about transcendental meditation

(1) It is easy to learn; there is no need to force the mind to do anything. During meditation the mind is allowed to reach a level of peace which is normally interfered with by other thought processes and outside distractions.
(2) It does not require the belief of any particular philosophy, the adherence to any religion, or indeed even a belief in TM itself, for it to be learnt and to be beneficial.

(3) It can be learnt by everyone, by men and women of all standards of intelligence and education and from all walks of life. TM is not only for the clever.
(4) The TM programme is quite safe, its benefits can be demonstrated objectively, the system of teaching is uniform, and the learning process is not altered by the beliefs or personality of the teacher.
(5) TM seeks to develop all the normal faculties of mind, body and emotions that we already possess. It therefore enables people to come nearer to their full potential as human beings.

The symptoms of ME appear to be greatly influenced by both mental and physical stress. In spite of the fact that we now know that the illness is triggered by a viral infection in most cases, and a virus seems to persist in the cells, there is another dimension to this illness, a psychological one.

It is true to say that *all* illness has a psychological dimension. Does prolonged mental stress cause physical symptoms? Or can prolonged physical symptoms, especially pain, cause mental distress? Who can really say which causes which, or what came first, and does it really matter?

To achieve physical rest one can lie on a bed or sit in a comfortable chair. It is far more difficult to rest mentally and emotionally.

Meditation is a technique for getting very high quality mental rest; but it is not only the mind that is quiet; TM produces a state of profound physiological rest of the body, at the same time as increasing mental alertness.

Mahareshi said (1960): 'I call it meditation, but it is in fact a technique of self exploration; it enables a man to dive into the innermost reaches of his being, in which dwell the essence of life and the source of all wisdom, all creativity, all peace, and all happiness. The word meditation is not new, nor are its benefits new, but for centuries the technique of this kind of meditation has been forgotten.'

Benefits of meditation

So what are the benefits of meditation to an ME patient?

In ME, there seems to be increased sensitivity to stress. The heart rate is raised, with palpitations, out of proportion to the stimulus of anxiety or minimal physical effort; the breathing is often disordered, with feelings of breathlessness, or of a weight on the chest; we have a tendency to nightmares, to unreasonable states of panic or anxiety, and to sleep disturbances.

We are constantly exhausted, sweat profusely, have unstable blood sugars; the circulation to hands and feet is often poor, and our thermostats don't work. We are excessively sensitive to noises, smells, touch, and pain, and over-react to situations.

Many of these symptoms are produced by being in a state of arousal resulting from fear, fright, anxiety, shock, or anticipation.

Some doctors at London's Charing Cross Hospital have assessed a group of patients with classic ME syndrome, some of whom had a positive blood test for enterovirus. The patients were found to be *overbreathing*, albeit quite unconsciously. The effects from this include 'twitchiness' of muscles, rapid heart beat, and lowered carbon dioxide in the blood.

Dr Peter Nixon, cardiologist at Charing Cross Hospital, has pioneered work for years on stress reduction and learning to breathe correctly, for patients with high blood pressure and heart disease. Looking at ME patients, he thought that the overbreathing 'was a symptom of fear or panic, that can be experienced by people who demand a lot of themselves and fall short in their achievements'.

In this research, some ME patients with overbreathing (hyperventilation) were admitted to hospital and sedated for several days, so that they slept most of the time. Not surprisingly, they all went home feeling better as a result of the prolonged sleep and total rest. They were also instructed in correct breathing, and had counselling to help them with a better insight into their problems. At the present time, there is no information about whether these patients maintained their improvement enough to live a normal life without relapsing.

However it is not disputed that once you develop ME, there is a strong chance that symptoms similar to constant stress arousal are present. Some of these unpleasant symptoms – pounding heart, sweating, diarrhoea, hypersensitivity to stimuli, feeling out of breath and panicky – may be due to disordered function of the master control nerve centres in the brain; this is the signal box which sets the light to '**danger**' and puts the body into a state ready for action, even though there is no danger. Or perhaps the symptoms are also due to the terrible uncertainty of not knowing for how long one is going to be unable to live a normal life, and by fighting the exhaustion.

Developing ME, for most sufferers, is far more stressful than the events preceding the illness. But whatever is causing the disordered state of the autonomic nervous system, be it due to the virus in the brain or due to unresolved fear and anxiety, or both, meditation has been found to help. How?

The effects of meditation have been extensively studied on subjects doing transcendental meditation, which is why this type of meditation is being quoted.

There are different techniques of meditating, and others may well have similar results.

Benefits resulting from transcendental meditation

(1) The physiological changes during the practice of TM indicate a state of quietness of the sympathetic nervous system, i.e. the opposite of the 'fight or flight' arousal state.
(2) During TM, the heart rate is decreased, the blood pressure is lowered, and the breathing rate is slower.
(3) Oxygen consumption by the whole body is reduced. In some studies oxygen consumption fell by up to 20 per cent during TM.
(4) There is an increase in blood flow to tissues. There is consequently better removal of waste products of metabolism and a lower level of lactic acid in the blood.
(5) During TM there is a decreased level of circulating cortisols. Long-term meditation is found to decrease resting cortisol levels even when not meditating.
(6) This reduction of adrenal gland activity is the opposite of Selye's stress response, and must be beneficial for ME.
(7) There is long-term stability of the autonomic nervous system through regular practice of TM.
(8) Research has demonstrated electro-encephalogram (EEG) changes during TM, which point to increased orderliness of brain functioning.
(9) Body reactions to loud noise are reduced, and there is improved temperature control.
(10) Gum inflammation was found to improve after TM – this may indicate a beneficial effect on the number and function of white cells. There has

been no research yet specifically on the effects of TM on the immune system, but by stress reduction one would expect the body's natural defences to become stronger.

There are various other effects of TM documented from research. It appears that many benefits are related to the regularity and length of time that TM is practised, particularly effects such as better motor co-ordination, better sleep, improved mental function, and overall better health.

There are other forms of meditation, but none have been so well researched as TM. Perhaps some people find other ways of meditation suit them better, there are no hard and fast rules about it. Meditation is not quite the same as relaxation techniques, or hypnotherapy, though physical relaxation, quieter breathing, slower pulse, and mental quietness should result from all these practices.

Teachers of TM can be found all over the world. The UK contact address is given in Appendix A.

Relaxation Techniques

There are classes for learning relaxation, and there are a great many relaxation tapes available. They range from simple instructions for physical relaxation, to guided imagery. Some are simply sounds of sea or music especially recorded over a quiet voice which is supposed to reach the unconscious.

The guided imagery is a voice which directs you to imagine yourself in some very beautiful tranquil place, and to experience this place vividly. This works well for some people. Others prefer to make their own tape, using their own voice, and using a description of a place which is known and special and has happy associations.

Suggested Further Reading

Anatomy of an Illness, by Norman Cousins (Bantam Books, 1979).

Getting Well Again, by Carl and Stephanie Simonton and James L. Creighton (Bantam Books, 1981).
(This book is written mainly for cancer patients, but is valid for everyone suffering from a chronic illness.)

Your Complete Stress Proofing Programme, by Leon Chaitow (Thorsons, 1985).

13

Low Blood Sugar (Hypoglycaemia)

Low blood sugar needs to be discussed in a book about ME, because some ME symptoms may be due to a drop in blood sugar levels; also because there may be people who, for various reasons, suffer from periodic low blood sugar but do not have ME.

Hypoglycaemia is easily overlooked as an easily treatable cause of many symptoms. It occurs:

(a) In insulin dependent *diabetics*, as a result of too much insulin, too little food, a delayed meal, sudden exercise – any condition of too little sugar to balance the injection insulin. Diabetics learn to recognize the early warning signals and to take preventative action by eating.

(b) In a very rare condition where there is a tumour of insulin producing cells of the pancreas. This is very serious and leads to profoundly low blood sugar levels, coma and possibly death.

(c) In people who for various reasons have a rapid fall in blood sugar levels between meals – called 'reactive hypoglycaemia' – this is the kind of problem we are looking at with ME or suspected ME patients.

    The symptoms result not only from the blood sugar being low, but also from a too rapid fall.

After a meal is eaten there is a steady rise in blood

sugar level as the food is digested and absorbed into the blood stream. This triggers off release of the sugar controlling hormone *insulin*, produced by certain cells in the pancreas. The insulin lowers blood sugar by pushing glucose into the cells; an untreated diabetic has loads of glucose in the blood, but is weak and exhausted because the body cells cannot use this glucose to burn to make energy, due to lack of insulin.

So in a healthy glucose balanced state, the blood levels are kept within upper and lower limits by the controlled insulin response, and there should be neither hyper not hypo-glycaemic symptoms.

Symptoms Produced by Rapid Fall in Blood Glucose

- Feeling faint or dizzy
- Nausea
- Sweating
- Pallor
- Rapid thin pulse
- Feeling 'spaced out'
- Irritability
- Irrational, bizarre behaviour (like someone drunk)
- Headache
- Poor concentration
- Inability to make decisions, panic attacks
- Slurred speech
- Blurred vision
- Fatigue, muscle weakness
- Unsteady gait
- Insomnia, waking in the night and not going back to sleep without eating.

Any of these symptoms may occur; the earliest

signs are hunger, faintness and inability to think straight. The commonest times are 11 a.m.–1 p.m. and 4–6 p.m., from two to four hours following a meal. If hunger itself is not present, then it may be easy to overlook hypoglycaemia as a cause of feeling unwell. If eating a meal banishes symptoms, this is further proof.

Many people who feel really ghastly first thing in the morning reach for a cup of coffee not just as a stimulant, but because caffeine boosts blood sugar – for a short time only. By 11 a.m. they are usually irritable and desperate for the next cup of coffee. Probably most accidents occur at work mid to late morning and late afternoon, and many road accidents may be caused by low blood sugar. How often do family rows flare up just before mealtimes?

We who live in wealthy countries have more than we need to eat, so how is it that hunger and low blood sugar cause so many people to feel unwell so much of the time? For this problem is extremely common, as any of you who have experienced the symptoms (even before getting ME) or who have irritable spouses and whining children at the end of the afternoon will know.

Most attacks of hypoglycaemia are rebound drops which follow a too rapid rise in blood sugar.

A *normal* blood sugar curve after a meal should look rather like Figure 1 on page 196.

An over-reactive, hypoglycaemic curve looks more like Figure 2.

Common Causes of Reactive Hypoglycaemia

(1) *Consumption of refined carbohydrates,* i.e. sugar, honey, sweets, chocolate, cakes, sweet drinks, white flour, etc.

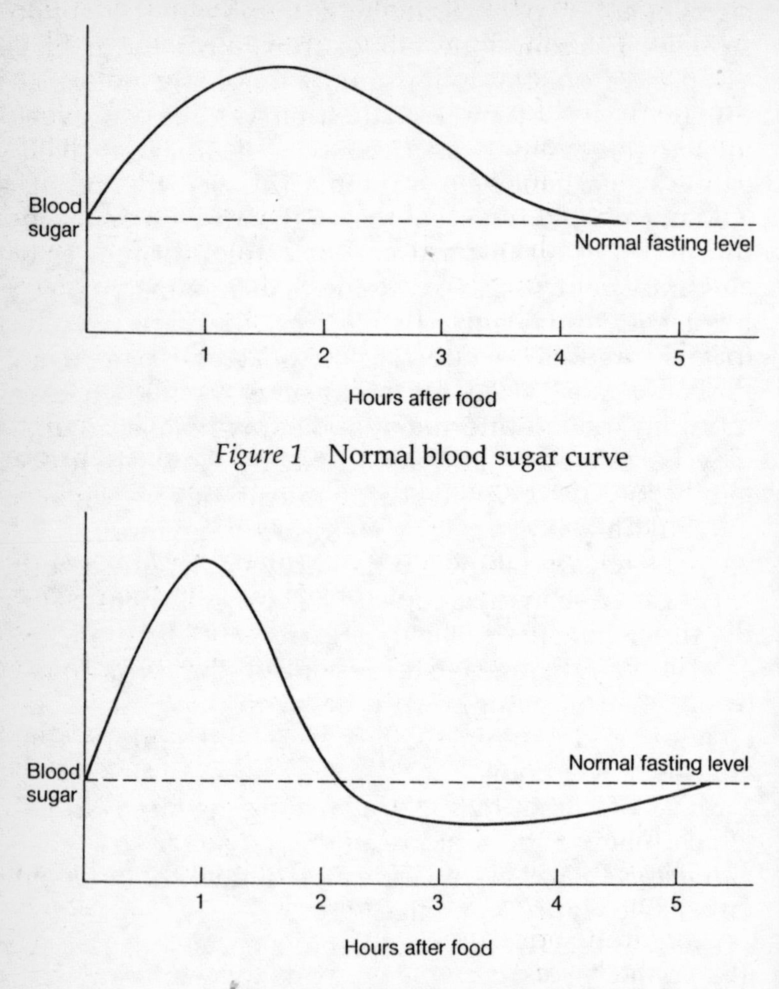

Figure 1 Normal blood sugar curve

Figure 2 Hypoglycaemic curve

This is *the* main dietary cause of hypoglycaemia, and has become worse with the advent of 'convenience' foods and with the trend towards eating snacks instead of balanced meals; the snacks so often consisting of buns, cakes, biscuits, chocolates or sweet bars, maybe washed down with coke or coffee with sugar in it. The result of these kinds of so-called 'foods' is a rapid rise in blood glucose, giving a temporary lift for an hour, followed by a rapid fall as insulin pours out from the pancreas in response to the sudden surge in sugar level.

So the binger on sweet things has violent swings in blood sugar through the day, with parallel mood changes. The long-term result of this can sometimes be pancreatic exhaustion and diabetes.

(2) *A reaction to an allergenic food*, e.g. wheat.

Hypoglycaemia may be a symptom of food allergies, and if the symptoms do not improve after following dietary advice for low blood sugar, then food allergy should be suspected.

(3) *Consumption of coffee, tea, alcohol.*

Caffeine and alcohol promote a rapid boost of blood sugar levels due to stimulating the release of sugar stored in the liver – followed by the rapid fall again. A large part of an alcoholic hangover is due to low blood sugar, the best cure for which is a hearty breakfast instead of coffee and aspirin. People who 'need' coffee or tea many times a day are reactive hypoglycaemics as well as caffeine addicts.

(4) *Nicotine* also stimulates a rise in blood sugar from liver reserves – no more need be said about cigarette addiction.

(5) *Candida yeast overgrowth* seems to lead to haywire sugar control. One theory proposed is that the yeast gobbles up the digested carbohydrate sugars preventing their absorption, but this is hard to prove. But anyway, those who improve on an anti-candida regime usually find their blood sugar control improves.

(6) *Stress*, such as anxiety, shock, grief, worry, over-

work, etc., is a potent factor in creating hypoglycaemia.

The reason is that when an alarm is triggered by some stress event, the body goes into a state of alertness for action or danger – the so-called 'fight or flight' response. Several things happen: the heart rate goes up, the blood pressure goes up, blood is diverted to muscles for instant action, sugar is mobilized from stores in liver and muscle into the circulation to provide rapid energy. In other words all systems are at GO; there is a state of excitement and anticipation.

Our hunting ancestors, people in combat and athletes use this state of alertness and dissipate all the energy by physical action. But the frustrated car driver, the harassed mother, the workaholic businessman at a desk, and the ME patient in a panic attack, do not use up these resources by physical action. Instead, their bodies stay at a constant level of stress reaction. This leads to lots of problems, including exhaustion and *low* blood sugar, because insulin comes along to lower the sugar level that was made ready for the physical activity that did not happen.

Any programme of management for hypoglycaemia needs to include some plan for stress reduction.

(7) *Hormonal disturbance.*

Many women find their sugar control worse in the ten days or so premenstrually, the hypoglycaemic symptoms contributing to the premenstrual tension and depression.

Too much or too little *thyroid* hormone may lead to low blood sugar, especially hypothyroidism (too little). This is because all hormones work together and affect each other, in a complicated delicately balanced manner, to maintain blood sugar and many other functions, in a stable state. An upset of any one has far reaching effects.

(8) *Nutritional deficiencies*.

A deficiency of vitamin B_6, *chromium*, zinc, manganese, magnesium, and other B vitamins can all increase the likelihood of hypoglycaemia. These nutrients are involved in the complicated chemical mechanisms mentioned above.

What is usually happening in someone with reactive hypoglycaemia is a combination of several or all of these factors.

Ways of Avoiding Hypoglycaemia

(1) *Eat regular meals*, if necessary eat four, five or six smaller meals instead of two or three per day. Try and stick to a regular pattern; the body clock comes to expect food at particular times, and delaying a meal by an hour or more can bring on symptoms.

(2) Eat a respectable breakfast, probably the most important meal of the day for a low blood sugar person. A cup of coffee and a slice of toast is not much to combat overnight starvation, yet millions of workers expect to get a morning's work done on just that. If you 'can't face food' on getting up, have some fruit and then something more substantial with protein at 9 or 10 a.m.

(3) Avoid sugars and refined starches completely. The answer to low blood sugar is *not* sugar, which perpetuates the problem, but is food which provides a more gradual sustained rise in

blood sugar, and does not stimulate the pancreas to throw out a sudden surge of insulin.

(4) Have either more protein with low carbohydrate meals, or have more complex carbohydrates. These are complete carbohydrates, unrefined, such as brown rice, wholemeal flour, wholegrains of all kinds, potatoes in skins.

For example, sugar free muesli for breakfast will provide more protein and roughage as well as carbohydrate, than cornflakes or white bread, and because it takes longer to be digested produces a more gradual sustained blood sugar rise.

(5) Fats delay absorption of food. The effect of a classic British breakfast of eggs and bacon tends to last all morning, as compared with cornflakes or toast. Bacon is not ideal, but eggs, or extra butter or marge, or a little pure vegetable oil mixed with muesli, may be helpful at breakfast.

(6) Have food available as snacks, but these should be sugar free, for example fresh nuts, cheese, Ryvita and peanut butter, a hard-boiled egg, cold meat, or wholemeal bread and spread other than jam or marmalade. Fruit may be acceptable, so long as it is not a kind with high sugar content.

(7) If you are a kitchen-raider at 3 a.m., have your evening meal later, or have a pre-bedtime mini-meal. A milky drink late evening can be helpful so long as milk is not a problem. Some ME people with this problem keep biscuits or crispbread or a sandwich ready on the bedside table at night.

(8) Avoid coffee, tea (except weak tea), cola, alcohol, and nicotine.

(9) If continued stress is a factor – and it seems to be

for many ME people – consider organizing some stress reduction.

Overbreathing is a frequent accompaniment to unrelieved stress and the 'fight or flight' arousal state. This can make hypoglycaemic symptoms worse, and increase the exhaustion of ME. Skilled help can correct this, and regimes such as yoga and meditation are very helpful.

(10) *Nutritional supplements*. The regime suggested on page 123 should provide all the necessary nutrients which are involved in blood sugar balance. It is worth taking a chromium supplement such as chromium GTF 200 micrograms daily, although a good multi-vitamin and mineral pill should contain some chromium. Chromium GTF supplementation, together with all B vitamins, has been found to balance both hypoglycaemia and diabetes. The best natural source is brewer's yeast, which is fine so long as it does not cause bloating or other candida symptoms.

The anti-stress nutrients, to protect against adrenal exhaustion, are: vitamin B_5 (pantothenic acid), vitamin B_3, magnesium, calcium, zinc, and vitamin C – so all these are important as well as chromium.

Not all people with ME have hypoglycaemia. Not all hypoglycaemics have ME. There is quite a lot of overlap in the symptoms, though, and the likelihood of having an unstable blood sugar seems to be greater among ME patients than the rest of the population. It seems sensible, whether or not you are diagnosed as having ME, to minimize hypoglycaemic attacks by following the above suggestions.

ME people most at risk of low blood sugar attacks

are those who *continue to do too much,* those who cannot reduce stress levels, and those who continue to eat poorly or infrequently.

14
Depression

There can be few ME victims who have not travelled down into the dark valley at some time during their illness. Depression is one of the commonest trials to be borne, and only those who have experienced real depression can truly sympathize with others so afflicted.

There is a difference between depression and unhappiness. The latter is usually the result of some bereavement, difficult circumstances, or perhaps the inability to adapt or come to terms with a situation. Other words used for such a feeling are sadness, dissatisfaction, 'feeling a bit blue', 'down in the dumps', or miserable.

Depression is an extension of the state of unhappiness beyond the point where the emotion can be explained by a cause. If someone grieves for a deceased loved one, their sadness is normal; but if the sadness continues for a long time after one would expect the grief to have settled, it may turn into depression.

Depression affects most bodily functions. The sleep pattern is usually disturbed, and it can be very distressing to wake in the night, alone with your black thoughts, unable to escape from them into sleep again. A depressed person may be cold and slow moving, the appetite is poor, there is lack of motivation, there may be slow or little speech, and constipation.

Worst of all is the feeling of isolation, that one is cut

off from other people and from experiencing any contact with beautiful things. An unhappy person may be moved to tears by beautiful music or a glorious sunset. A really depressed person will hear or see such things and feel absolutely nothing except perhaps despair because the contact with them is gone.

With depression there is commonly lack of motivation, insight, or judgement. The general purposelessness of life for the sufferer is seen in cruel contrast to the apparent industry and contentment of other people.

The really awful thing about depression is that you hate being in the blackness but cannot climb out of it. Well-meaning friends suggest that you snap out of it, or read a good book; that you should think of the world's starving children, and many such excellent remedies. But when you feel so very low, you often cannot read, or concentrate on the radio, or even speak on the phone.

Why is Depression so Common in ME?

(1) All *virus infections* cause some degree of depression.

(2) *Interferon* is one of the chemicals which help to limit a virus infection. When interferon was used to treat patients for another virus, the side effects complained of were fatigue, muscle aches and depression. So it has been postulated that many ME symptoms may be caused by continued production of interferon in the body as a response to a persistent virus.

(3) If the virus takes up residence in some brain cells and disrupts their function, then quite a lot of

brain functions are interfered with. Transmission of impulses between nerve cells takes place via chemical messengers, called neuro-transmitters. The neuro-transmitters that are known are derived from amino acids.

Amino acid	*Neuro-transmitter*
phenylalanine }	noradrenaline
tyrosine }	+ dopamine
tryptophan	serotonin
histidine	histamine
glutamic acid	GABA
+ vitamin B_6	

The chemical reactions also need various enzymes in order to work.

Therefore a lack of any of the amino acids or of enzymes leads to a deficiency of one or more neuro-transmitters, and this can greatly affect mood. Most of the drugs used to influence mood work by altering the level of neuro-transmitters.

For example, too little circulating noradrenaline can lead to depression. The 'tricyclic' anti-depressants increase noradrenaline levels.

The neuro-transmitter called GABA is an inhibitor of nerve functions, it *calms down* nervous reactions. A lack of vitamin B_6 (pyridoxine), which is needed to make GABA, is associated with increased tension, twitching, irritability, convulsions, and pins and needles.

These names and examples have been given to show that depression, and other mood changes such as manic behaviour, anxiety, and even schizophrenia, usually result from chemical changes in the parts of the brain concerned with behaviour and emotions.

No one has invented a way of doing a biopsy on these parts of the brain on a living person. So, unlike muscle fibres in ME which can be chopped out and looked at with an electron microscope, brain cells affected by a virus retain their secrets, and we don't understand exactly what is going wrong. So ME depression is very often an expression of the persistent virus infection playing havoc with brain cells and enzymes and neuro-transmitters.

The depression should therefore be seen as yet another nasty *symptom*, rather than to do with the personality of the sufferer. Many ME sufferers are people with no previous history of depression, and their behaviour can change alarmingly with ME. Uncontrollable tears, terrible black depression, despair, panic, suicidal thoughts – all these can be felt by someone previously regarded as well-adjusted and in control of their emotions. Such a miserable wreck can also become cheerful, laughing, or manic, this transformation taking place overnight or even within a day. All these emotional ups and downs are quite bewildering to both sufferers and those around them.

The depression that has been discussed above is a true *organic depression*, and is a feature of other diseases as well as ME; it is commonly associated with hormone disturbances such as low thyroid or adrenal function, in malnutrition, and chronic infections.

There is also an element of *reactive depression* in ME. The realization that you have an illness, which effectively puts a stop to most activities which you used to do, is enough to make anyone unhappy. You actually grieve for the person you were before you became ill. This loss is not unlike that of someone who retires or is made redundant after many active years in a fulfilling job. There is inevitably a sense of not being needed; the world carries on very well without you, a world in which we are judged by what we are seen to do and achieve. You grieve for the loss of the gardener, the athlete, the superhuman caring mother, the good cook, the cricketer, or the person who always had time for others – for all the different skills you had and things you enjoyed doing.

You react, too, to the prospect of possibly being disabled; to crossing over to join a society of people who were once 'them', not 'us'. And being disabled, when you look fairly normal to the onlooker, can lead to disbelief and lack of help from others. ME sufferers who cannot walk far do not have a large plaster cast which proclaims, 'See, I have broken my leg.'

And then part of the reaction to finding yourself ill with ME is naturally anger. One view of depression is that it is anger turned inside. Of course you are angry at getting ME, and at such a very inconvenient time, when there is so much you were planning to do. Because one is flattened, inactive, and maybe inarticulate, the anger is overlooked and very often suppressed.

Expressing anger in a constructive way is often used as part of psychotherapy for all sorts of mental problems; however if you are flat on your back and saving your energy to do essential things like eating and going to the bathroom, you will not feel like hitting pillows or shouting to vent your rage. Some people are angry with themselves, especially if they are led to believe that they have developed ME through doing too much, or that they are paying the price for mistakes made along life's path. You would be surprised to know how many people feel guilty about being ill. In spite of knowing about external causes of disease, the primitive belief that sickness may be some sort of retribution brought on oneself, does exist, though not openly admitted.

If you are angry, and then angry with yourself, and the anger persists inside, after a time you dislike yourself. Depression is a form of loss of self-esteem. If you have ME and depression, the loss of self-esteem is unfortunately reinforced by the loss of ability to work or function normally.

So there are two main causes of depression, one is the chemical imbalance in the brain due to the virus interfering with normal brain cell function, the other is the reaction of anger and grief at developing ME.

There are other factors which may, if present, tip the scales between just coping and becoming depressed. These are:

- *Exhaustion*, which may precede a relapse;
- *Low blood sugar*, which is treatable;
- *Candida overgrowth* – there are probably other symptoms to suggest this;
- *Hormonal changes*, for example premenstrual depression;
- *A food allergy* reaction;
- Reaction to some unsuspected *chemical*, for example gas central heating switched on;
- Some *personal upset*, loss of someone's affection, or other of life's emotional hazards;
- *Occasions* like Christmas, which make many people depressed especially if they are lonely or ill;
- *Dark winter* days.

It would be wonderful if one could slip into a safe coat of armour as soon as the early warning signs of depression appear. People who have been into the black pit and have come out again, and most do come out, can usually recognize when they are going down again. Before the thing has got hold of you and you don't have the will or insight to sort anything out, try looking to see if there is any factor tipping you over, which you can maybe change, or at least comprehend.

Early Stage of Depression Checklist

- Are you overdoing things? Extra rest and sleep, and letting go of striving, may help.
- Are you eating enough and of the right things?
- If you are female, is your period due soon? If so, you know this bad bout will not last for ever. Premenstrual depression is very common with women with ME, and may respond to extra vitamin B_6, magnesium, evening primrose oil, frequent meals and extra rest.
- If you have had symptoms pointing to candida overgrowth, could you be having a flare up, and need to take nystatin and check your diet?
- Have you eaten something you normally avoid to which you may be hypersensitive, such as wheat? If so, this reaction will pass.
- Is there some extra chemical around, such as gas or new paint? If you cannot avoid it, take extra vitamin C and wait for the reaction to settle, or consider going away.
- Is it a time of year when you have felt bad before? Many sufferers seem to find a seasonal pattern to their ups and downs. There is not much you can do about the earth turning, but at least you know it will go on turning and bring you to a better month. If it is winter, maybe a full spectrum lamp will help if you cannot get outside.
- Weather can also influence mood. Usually this does not last for very long, either. Damp weather seems to affect a lot of people, maybe because of

an associated increase of moulds and fungal spores in the air.

- Is your low mood the result of some personal upset? If so, try and talk about it to someone you trust, instead of bottling it up.

This list of things which may trigger off a depression may be of no use at all to you. Unfortunately, you can think that ME is receding, or that you have really got this illness sorted out and are coping *wonderfully* (so friends may think), when crash, down you go into the black pit, and absolutely nothing you do seems to pull you out.

There you are again, paralysed, weighed down by the big black bird that is there every morning when you wake after a fitful escape into sleep.

When I went through a very bad patch, I thought about putting myself out of my and everyone else's misery. I tried funny books but the words made no sense. I got a friend to take me to church, but I couldn't bear to see all those normal devout people whom God probably loved, and I was too ill to sit in a cold hard pew anyway. I looked at primroses and felt no wonder at their existence, only bitterness that things were growing and developing and I was apparently shrinking. I felt totally cut off from other human experience as though I was encased in a bubble that kept other people's love away from me.

I expect all this is familiar to many people with ME. I used to try and blot out the awfulness by taking sleeping pills in the vain hope of sleeping all night and waking up better. But the big black bird was still there at 2 a.m. and never went away.

Coping with Depression

So what encouragement can be offered to a really depressed ME sufferer? Well the big black bird *does* go away in time; mine left me, I could not be writing this if it was still there.

The following ideas may help carers as well as patients, and if you have ME and are at present well enough to read and understand this, then store this information up against a future bad time.

Remember that you, a unique special person, are the same person underneath the depression. Try to hold on to this fact, that the essential *you*, your spirit and soul, is intact, even when you feel disintegrated and cut off from the world. Try to see the depression as an awful thing to be borne patiently until it passes.

This time of blackness will pass. Be very patient with yourself, remember that seasons come and go and so do moods.

Do not feel ashamed of being as you are. If you have a persistent virus playing havoc in your body, you are allowed to have spells of depression just as much as spells of nausea or muscle pain. It's much harder to cope with, though.

Make a list (on paper, or in your head) of all the people you have ever known who like you, love you, or care about what happens to you. Do this while you are less depressed, and take this list out and refer to it if you have a bad time. Those people *still* care about you while you are depressed.

Allow those people who love you to give you their affection even if you cannot give anything back at the time. The thoughts and prayers of others can sustain you during a long bad patch. Michael Mayne, the present Dean of Westminster and an ME sufferer, said, 'When I was depressed I found I could not even pray, so I had to allow others to do the praying for me.'

Some of you may live alone, and say that you have no one who cares about you. There is probably someone, maybe at a distance, who could be contacted by phone or a written note. Could any friend fail to respond to a simple plea? Something like: 'I'm going through a very bad patch just now – please think of me, or phone me, or come and see me.'

The majority of those other people out there who appear to be happy and stable have probably gone through depression at some time in their lives. Those most able to understand and give support are those who have been in the dark valley and know what it is like. Such people may be contactable through your local ME support group or local church, or telephone the Samaritans.

As far as circumstances allow and you are able, pamper yourself, give yourself treats. Or allow others to give you treats. This could vary from a nice warm bath with essential oils in it, a new soft nightgown, something very good to eat, or a visit from a hairdresser and some make-up; to an outing in a car to a lovely place, a new book or record, some beautiful flowers, etc. A big problem of course is that if you have depression *and* ME, you will probably not be physically up to outings in the car or a nice concert. An outing to sit in a comfortable chair in a garden or covered verandah might be more appropriate.

One of the classic features of a depression is the loss of self-esteem. By trying to give yourself treats, you are reinforcing your affection for yourself. There is nothing wrong with loving yourself. Loving yourself is not the same as selfishness, it means accepting and caring about your individual personality with all its faults and weaknesses, just as you accept the weaknesses and imperfections of a friend or loved one.

Try looking in a mirror, and saying to the face in it (no matter if it looks a bit haggard just now), 'You are really very nice underneath that picture of misery. I like you and want you to get better', or words to that effect. It may seem so incongruous that it is funny. Anything that can seem funny is a good thing when you are down, even if it is only your own woebegone reflection.

One way to boost self-esteem is to manage to complete a small task each day. Now there is no point in setting impossible goals that no self-respecting ME person could achieve without collapse, so the task needs to be something within your grasp.

Writing one or more short letters or notes, sewing on a button, turning out some drawers or a desk, or doing a small patch of weeding, according to your ability at the time. The positive feedback from accomplishing something, especially if you see the result, as in mending or tidying, can give a small boost each day.

A certain degree of apathy may need to be overcome, but it is amazing how once the initial effort is made, the concentration required can sometimes overcome the darkness for a time.

But do not set a goal which is beyond your powers; if the task is unreasonable, you will give up half-way through and this can be counterproductive.

What about Anti-Depressants?

Anti-depressants, like all drugs, may be unsuitable for some ME sufferers who are very sensitive to many medicines.

It might be worth trying tryptophan, an amino acid

precursor of serotonin, a neuro-transmitter which influences mood. Tryptophan also has mildly sedative properties, and 500 mg to 1,000 mg taken in the evening can help with insomnia as well as depression. It is normally taken about 500 mg twice daily, morning and evening to start with, if being used to treat depression. This can be gradually increased to up to 2 grams three times a day, under medical supervision. Improvement in mood and sleeping usually happens within seven to ten days.

The other amino acid that may help depression is phenylalanine, the precursor of noradrenaline. Sometimes tryptophan is used together with other anti-depressants in severe depression.

Anti-depressants have helped many ME sufferers. Others have been unable to tolerate them, or have found no benefit. There is no absolute rule about this form of therapy. What I think is very interesting, though, is that some patients have found that their ME as a whole has improved from anti-depressant treatment. Does this mean then that ME is a psychiatric illness, and the physical symptoms are secondary to the mental problem?

No, ME is still an organic disease that affects all parts of the body.

The anti-depressants called tricyclics (because of their chemical formula) were originally developed as antihistamines to treat allergies. It was noticed that patients receiving them felt much better in their mood, so they came to be used to treat depression; other chemicals were developed as the antihistamines used today.

The chemical formulae of the tricyclics, the antihistamines used to treat hay fever and skin allergies,and the phenothiazines used to treat schizophrenia and mania, are very similar. In fact tricyclic anti-depressants are sometimes used to treat chronic skin problems.

Tricyclics work by altering the available levels of some neuro-transmitters, with effects not only on mood, but on the transmission of other nerve impulses. So it is not surprising that brain functions in general improve, such as memory, concentration, sleep patterns, and sensitivity to pain and noise. As this drug also has antihistamine effects, it would modify some allergic symptoms as well. And moreover, some ME patients say their muscle weakness and pain also improved with tricyclics. In theory, this sounds like a wonder drug for ME!

The commonsense conclusion from the above is to say to an ME patient who is not getting better, and has tried diet, vitamins, candida treatment and some treatment of any stress:

Do not dismiss anti-depressants if your doctor suggests this treatment. Don't throw away the chance of something that may help, just because it is called 'anti-depressant'. We are so keen for the world to recognize our illness as real and not based on neurosis, that we tend to shy away from any treatment which smells of psychiatry! It would be better to call these medicines tricyclics, or mono-amine-oxidase inhibitors (MAOIs – this is the other main group) instead of anti-depressants.

Sadly, there is a small but steady toll of people with ME who find they just cannot bear life any more, and take the only route left to them.

Perhaps they would not have commited suicide **if** they had had someone who believed and supported them; **if** they had a sympathetic employer; **if** they had seen a doctor aware enough to place them under supervision and start anti-depressant treatment before it was too late.

So **please**, if you as an ME sufferer, or someone you know, is seriously depressed and has thought or talked of suicide, **do get medical help**, and don't refuse treatment or short-term hospital admission if this is advised. These tragedies are avoidable.

Not everyone will consider tricyclic drugs. Some may find their depression is helped by a nutritious diet, plus extra B vitamins, zinc and magnesium, and perhaps tryptophan or a total amino acid supplement. If anti-depressants are prescribed, then those with the least side effects should be used, and starting with the smallest dose.

Some have sedative properties, others are less sedative and more stimulating. In New Zealand, some doctors are finding that a tricyclic called Prothiaden – chemical name is dothiepin – seems to work best.

There are some which are slightly modified, called quadricyclics. Examples of these are mianserin and maprotiline – these are their chemical names; trade names may differ in different countries, e.g. Ludiomil, Bolvidon. (Who thinks up these names?)

The important thing to remember about anti-depressants is that they do not work overnight like aspirins or sleeping pills. It will be at least two weeks before you see any real improvement in mood. Before that, most people benefit from better sleep and less anxiety, a great relief if there is marked insomnia and agitation as well as depression.

Side effects

Possible *side effects* from tricyclics are:

> Dry mouth, blurred vision, difficulty passing urine, constipation, low blood pressure, dizziness, irregular or slow heart beats.

Most side effects settle after the first week or two, especially if the dose is increased gradually.

The starting dose should be much smaller for an ME sufferer than for others.

For example, Prothiaden 25 mg at night, gradually increasing to 100 to 150 mg, or Trimiprimine 10 mg at night, increasing to 75 mg or more daily.

If you have unpleasant side effects at the start of treatment, especially any heart symptoms or missed beats, tell your doctor. ME patients who have palpitations or other heart symptoms, and bladder problems, should be sure to mention these to their doctor if anti-depressants are considered. Some of the newer tricyclics and the quadricyclics have fewer of the side effects listed above.

The other main type of anti-depressants, MAOIs, should not be used as first choice, unless for very good reason. They interact with any foods that contain tyramine or other amines, and alarming rises in blood pressure can happen. If you are put on MAOIs you will be given a list of all the dangerous foods, which include cheese and broad beans. This is one more hazard for an ME patient to contend with – life is complicated enough without yet more foods to avoid.

Treatment is usually continued for at least a month after symptoms improve, before there is any attempt to reduce the dose.

If you are getting better on anti-depressants **do not suddenly stop them**. Even if you feel cheerful and think you don't need them any more, you need to reduce the daily dose very gradually under regular medical supervision. Sudden withdrawal could put you right back to where you started from or even worse.

If you are not taking any nutritional supplements

already, consider the following, all of which are necessary for good brain function:

vitamins B_1, B_6, nicotinic acid (B_3) and B_{12} – best taken as a yeast free B complex which has at least 20 mg of vitamin B_6
vitamin C
zinc
magnesium

Psychotherapy

This sounds rather alarming, and may suggest that the patient is mentally unsound and needs sorting out.

The term is used here rather loosely, and refers to the sort of skilled help that can be given by a psychiatrist, a psychotherapist, a counsellor, or anyone else trained in this field.

It is not suggested for someone in the early acute stage of illness, nor during a relapse, because there just is not the energy available for the talking and self-understanding that is part of the therapy.

One of the main steps to take before you can cope with any chronic illness is to accept the illness and come to terms with the limitations it imposes; and some time spent with a skilled counsellor may help to achieve this acceptance.

Psychotherapy in the accepted sense is much too strenuous for someone with ME to attempt. To be done properly it may involve a year or more of commitment to sessions lasting from one to two hours, and the process can be quite painful emotionally even to someone in good physical health.

Anger and grief are perfectly normal reactions to

developing a condition such as ME. If these emotions can be expressed and admitted, instead of being suppressed and driven inside, then the sufferer has a better chance of maintaining a degree of sanity, and of coping with further relapses or depression.

Often, family and friends really want to help the ME sufferer, whom they see is devastated by the symptoms and loss of normal life, but they may not have the skills needed to help psychologically. So seeing an outsider who has these skills is worth thinking about when you are not acutely ill or starting a relapse.

Loneliness

I have talked about grief and anger and their role in contributing to depression. Loneliness is an emotion that hurts a lot of ME people, even those living in a family situation. Chronic illness may lose you friends, but it need not; a lot depends on how you view your friends and family. For example, if you become jealous of the health of others, this shows and drives them away. Self-pity, moaning about how unfair life is, and seeing yourself as a victim all lead in the end to resentment. These emotions get between you and friends and lead to loneliness.

Past hurts and grievances, if they are hung on to, eat away inside and also cause resentment. All sorts of barriers that stop you loving other people and keep their affection from you can spring up from jealousy and resentment.

Loneliness is partly a state of mind. People can feel lonely surrounded by a crowd in a city, or not feel lonely while apparently isolated in a deserted landscape. The key to this is being content with yourself, liking yourself enough to want to have *you* as your friend.

Here are some words of the writer Kahlil Gibran, taken from his little masterpiece *The Prophet*. They speak clearly about unhappiness and the pain of depression.

> ... *Of Joy and Sorrow* ...
> When you are joyous, look deep into your heart and you shall find it is only that which has given you sorrow that is giving you joy.
>
> When you are sorrowful, look again in your heart, and you shall see that in truth you are weeping for that which has been your delight.
>
> Some of you say, 'Joy is greater than sorrow', and others say, 'Nay, sorrow is the greater'.
>
> But I say unto you, they are inseparable.
>
> Together they come, and when one sits alone with you at your board, remember that the other is asleep upon your bed.
>
> ... *Of Pain* ...
> Your pain is the breaking of the shell that encloses your understanding.
>
> Even as the stone of the fruit must break, that its heart may stand in the sun, so must you know pain.
>
> And could you keep your heart in wonder at the daily miracle of your life, your pain would not seem less wondrous than your joy;
>
> And you would accept the seasons of your heart, even as you have always accepted the seasons that pass over your fields.
>
> And you would watch with serenity through the winters of your grief.

15

Daylight and Oxygen

This chapter is being written in a greenhouse. It is mid July in England, it is pouring with rain and there is no likelihood of the sun appearing today to make the temperature in here intolerable. Moving in to the greenhouse became desirable because it was dark inside the house, also I had a bad headache and a craving for fresh air. Amazingly, in here there is full daylight; the tomato plants, lawn and trees provide a refreshing green background, and the air seems soft and full of oxygen. (This is a greenhouse in which there are no sprays or chemicals of any kind.) It seems an appropriate environment in which to discuss the benefits of light and oxygen to an ME sufferer – it has also cleared the headache.

The natural daylight seems far better for tired eyes than the electric light that was switched on in the house. Looking at the rows of tomato plants reminds me of plant physiology, that in daylight, green plants take in carbon dioxide and give off oxygen, so perhaps the good feeling in here is not just psychological.

Before you rush off to set up a settee or sunbed in a greenhouse or conservatory, please ensure that there are no pots or tins of chemicals or fertilizers around, and that the door or window is open. Bear in mind as well that on days when the sun does shine, it can reach 100°F under glass! Then it is better to move the bed/chair outside in the shade.

Seriously, though, natural daylight and sunshine are extremely important for health; not only because of the skin making vitamin D in daylight, nor because of the undoubted psychological boost it gives, but because full spectrum light entering the eyes has a direct effect on health.

There are various behavioural patterns, seen in animals and plants, which result from changes in light. These include migration, hibernation, stimulus for courtship and breeding, sleep and activity, growth, and opening or closing of leaves and petals, to name a few.

Light exerts a profound effect on plants and all animal life. We humans have largely overcome life-style restrictions due to natural darkness through the invention of electric light. Before electric light, there were oil lamps, candles and gas lamps, but these sources of light had limitations and probably did not influence our way of life to the extent that electricity has. With electric light, people can stay awake as late as they like, can work all day without daylight, and in fact there are few activities for which our forefathers depended on light, which cannot now take place in artificial light.

Dr John Ott, an American scientist, studied the effects of different kinds of light on plants, animals and humans in the 1960s and 1970s. In his book, *Health and Light*, he described the difference in the health and size of mink in breeding sheds, where one shed received light reflected off an aluminium wall, while the others had light reflected off corrugated iron.

The animals in the shed next to the aluminium wall were healthier, larger, and had greater numbers of young than in the other sheds, although other factors such as temperature, food, water and cage size were identical. Using an ultraviolet light meter, Dr Ott found that there were decidedly higher levels of ultraviolet light being reflected into the area where the mink had been doing very well.

Talking of the loss of light from air pollution in cities, Dr Ott wrote,

> The loss of 10 to 14 percent of visible sunlight and even more of ultraviolet is frightening, but civilized man has cut himself off from much greater percentages of sunlight by living indoors behind walls and glass.
>
> He has developed artificial sources of illumination that are gross distorters of the visible light spectrum of natural sunlight and almost totally devoid of any ultraviolet. The number of people wearing glasses and contact lenses is increasing; even when they are outdoors, most ultraviolet is being blocked from their eyes. Dark sunglasses and tinted lenses cause further light pollution. To what extent is this artificial or polluted light environment affecting man's health and well being?

John Ott also records how he himself suffered badly from arthritis, at a time when he was spending a lot of time inside recording studios, participating in time-sequence movie shots of plants. He accidentally broke his glasses, and spent some days outside in sunlight, being unable to drive or to work without them. To his surprise, his arthritic pains improved dramatically, but worsened if he had to spend time again inside or behind glass. He had previously rested lying in sunlight, wearing sunglasses, with no benefit to the arthritis at all. He found that the easing of the pain only took place when he exposed his eyes to full spectrum light, outside, several hours a day without glass lenses in front of his eyes.

There is a group of people who suffer from depression each winter, but not during the rest of the year; their depression is seasonally related, probably to the amount of daylight. I do not know if their mental symptoms would improve if they tried to spend several hours a day in daylight outside glass or buildings; probably no one has suggested this.

The mechanisms whereby exposure to full spectrum daylight affects mood, health, well-being, and fertility (in animals) has not been fully investigated. It is known that the influence of light depends largely on an adequate level of the ultraviolet part of the visible spectrum being received in the eyes. There are direct nerve connections between photoreceptive cells in the retina of the eye, and the pineal gland, which is a small outgrowth of the brain situated behind the hypothalamus, deep within the brain.

The pineal is probably involved in co-ordinating circadian and diurnal rhythms in different organs of the body, doing this by way of the hypothalamus and pituitary gland. It seems to be an active gland, and probably secretes hormones into the circulation to affect other parts of the brain or body; so it could well have some influence on general health, probably via other hormone secreting glands.

Many ME sufferers have reported a deterioration from November through till the spring. It is possible that one of the factors responsible is a relative lack of light, although there may be others, such as cold and damp, and increased exposure to various heating fumes and other indoor pollution.

Nevertheless, we should remember that in tuberculosis sanatoriums, in the bad days before streptomycin and other anti-TB drugs came into being, very ill patients on long-term bed rest were put outside on open verandahs all the year round, so they could receive the benefits of both fresh air and sunlight.

I am not suggesting that people with ME, who are frequently light sensitive, should sit outside and try and look directly at the sun! But it does make sense to get outside each day if you are well enough; in strong sunlight sit or lie in the shade, for there is plenty of good light reflected around even when sitting out of direct sunlight. Someone virtually bedridden should at least spend some time by a window with sunlight; even though glass cuts out some light, it is better than nothing. If you wear glasses, leave them off while sitting or resting outside. If it is bright, the eyes can be closed, light still enters through the lids.

It may be worth investing in a lamp which emits the complete range of light, to use in a bedroom if you are bed-bound for some time. The best places to look for these are garden centres, where they are supplied to give full spectrum light for sensitive plants in winter.

Fresh Air and Oxygen

Unpolluted air to breathe is desirable for everyone. The oxygen is essential, but there are very many unwanted substances in the air that can damage lungs, affect brains of children, especially lead from car exhausts, and make chemically sensitive people ill. Fortunately the air in most major cities has improved in quality following the Clean Air Act and the introduction of smoke-free zones.

But the visible smoke and smog from thousands of coal burning homes have been replaced by ever increasing pollution from petrol and diesel fumes, as more and more people use motor cars to travel even quite short distances. In Tokyo the toxicity is so bad in the city centre that traffic policemen have to change over after less than half an hour.

Pollution is just as bad inside many buildings, because of the increased use of plastic and foam-based furnishings and equipment, 'air conditioning' which may recirculate dust and germs, and many different sprays, paints and so-called air fresheners.

But apart from pollution, what about oxygen? It is present in a concentration of about 20 per cent in all air, is taken into the lungs with each breath, and is distributed round the body to every living cell, carried in red blood cells.

Oxygen supply of some tissues in ME seems to be poor, especially during a relapse. There are several possible reasons for this:

- The circulation to the extremities (hands and feet) is poor; complaints of cold hands and toes, which may turn white, blue, or even nearly black, are common even in summer.
- The muscle tone in small arteries may be faulty, interfering with the normally smooth flow of blood and elasticity of vessel walls after each pulse from the heart beat.
- The small blood vessels may be too constricted due to faulty nerve impulses from the brain via the autonomic nervous system.
- In some cases there may be a reduced blood flow in small vessels due to reduced heart output, if the heart muscle is affected, as in myocarditis.
- There seems to be some disorder of breathing regulation, especially at night. Tests on ME patients in a sleep laboratory have shown that there are periods during sleep when a patient stops breathing for a minute or so, called 'apnoea' periods. This may explain why some have the alarming symptom of waking up feeling short of

breath, and need to sit up and take some deep breaths. I do not know why this happens.

- Breathing at rest is controlled by the respiratory centre in the brain. This responds to levels of carbon dioxide (mainly) and oxygen in the blood. Perhaps this vital part of the brain is also affected by the ME syndrome. There is, however, no danger of stopping breathing for a dangerously long time.
- It is probable that, during a relapse, there is something wrong with the red blood cells, making it harder for them to travel along the smallest vessels (capillaries) to supply oxygen to tissues. Researchers in Australia have examined the blood of patients with the classic features of ME, during and after relapse. The red blood cells were seen to become abnormally shaped during a relapse, losing their bi-concave, smooth, disc-like appearance. In this form, red cells would be less able to pass through capillaries. This odd appearance had only been observed before in red blood cells of athletes who had just run a marathon.

  These findings would explain the poor microcirculation and poor oxygenation of tissues, and hence impaired removal of by-products of metabolism such as lactic acid from muscles.

Preliminary trials of increasing oxygen supply to ME patients have shown some benefit. The procedure is to supply oxygen via a small nasal tube during sleep. Research on this is starting at a London hospital, and although at this time the trials are not completed, most patients having oxygen therapy report some benefit. For those who are very ill, especially with symptoms of bad circulation, or evidence of poor oxygenation of the tissues, it may (in the UK) be possible to have an oxygen supply on loan from the NHS, to use at night; the oxygen is delivered through a nasal catheter.

It makes sense for any ME person who feels 'oxygen starved' to do some deep breathing twice a day outside or by an open window. Rooms should be well-ventilated as well as warm; there are various ways of improving breathing techniques, including yoga.

By yoga I do not necessarily mean standing on your head, or indeed any of the advanced postures. There are some good self-teaching books around, which can show you the basic breathing and very simple posture techniques. Yoga improves breathing, circulation and oxygen supply to tissues.

Hyperbaric Oxygen Therapy

There is a possibility that treatment by hyperbaric oxygen may be of benefit to some ME sufferers. At the present time only a few have tried this. The treatment involves breathing oxygen under pressure, sitting in a large chamber along with some other patients. This results in an increased oxygen partial pressure in the blood, with improved delivery of oxygen to the tissues.

Hyperbaric oxygen therapy has been used for some years by people with multiple sclerosis. Treatment chambers are available at various Action for Research into Multiple Sclerosis (ARMS) treatment centres around the country.

No clinical trials of this kind of oxygen therapy have been carried out for ME patients yet. In theory it should be helpful for many symptoms of ME which are associated with poor oxygenation of tissues and problems of cell membrane function, such as muscle pains, poor brain function and energy levels. It is unlikely to hasten the departure of a persistent virus. It is hoped that more will be learned about this therapy and ME in due course.

Meanwhile, if any ME sufferer wishes to find out more about hyperbaric oxygen therapy, or to try it, they can contact ARMS for information, and location of treatment centres. (Address in Appendix A.)

16

Drugs, Dentistry, Immunizations

ME patients need to be very cautious about taking medicines for various reasons; so many sufferers become hypersensitive to drugs, and in some there may be a problem in breakdown and disposal of a drug if the liver is at all affected. Drugs affecting the nervous system may produce quite bizarre effects, sometimes the opposite of what is intended.

A good rule is to discuss with your doctor any medicine you may be prescribed. You need to know exactly what it is – its name and purpose, the symptoms it is supposed to treat, how to take it, and how long for. Report any possible side effects as soon as possible. Various self-medications which can be bought at a chemist's, and were once harmless, may now cause side effects or allergy reactions if you have ME. Beware of medicines or pills that have colourings which cause a reaction, and be aware that many cough medicines also contain sugar or alcohol. If in doubt, ask the pharmacist what is in any liquid medicine, and avoid preparations that are highly coloured.

Drugs to be avoided if at all possible include:

Tranquillizers (e.g. Valium, Librium, Ativan).
These can be addictive, can make depression worse, and do not do anything to correct underlying brain disturbance.

Antibiotics – especially broad spectrum ones.
Ideally, proof of a bacterial infection should be obtained first, such as a urine culture for suspected bladder or kidney infection, or throat swab for tonsillitis; and if an antibiotic is deemed as essential, hopefully your doctor will prescribe one specifically for that infection, for a limited length of time. The sensible ME patient who develops an infection will take measures to help the white blood cells overcome it, such as extra vitamin C (up to 9 gm daily), zinc, vitamin A, extra rest and plenty of fluids.

If you require a course of antibiotics, take the complete course; a half-hearted course leads to more trouble as the germs may come back, and may develop resistance to that antibiotic. Restore the friendly bugs in your gut, which will have been depleted by the antibiotic, by taking probiotics for at least two weeks after the antibiotics are finished. (See page 137).

Steroids
If you are already taking cortico-steroids, i.e. cortisone, prednisolone, ACTH, or something similar, **do not stop taking them**, but consult your GP or specialist about the need for them. Unfortunately, steroids may cause temporary improvement of symptoms in many conditions, including asthma, multiple sclerosis, arthritis, bowel conditions such as ulcerative colitis and Crohn's disease, polymyalgia and many others.

The dramatic improvement happens because the body's own supply of cortisone is boosted artificially; this can dampen down the symptoms which result from allergic reactions (e.g. asthma), or from the immune system's recognition of self from non-self getting confused and reacting with own tissues – the so-called 'auto-immune' diseases.

Short-term benefits are outweighed by the longer-term effects of steroids: laziness of the adrenal-cortex glands in making one's own cortisone, leading to poor response to stress and infection, and to increasing dependence on the steroid drug as the source of cortisone. Also the suppression of symptoms does nothing to correct the underlying problem which produced them. It may also mask other serious conditions such as TB or cancer. Natural cortisone levels fluctuate during 24 hours; this natural response to the body's needs cannot be duplicated by regular pills. Other side effects can be high blood pressure, fluid retention, loss of calcium from bones leading to osteoporosis, muscle weakness, diabetes, stomach ulcers and mental problems – maybe serious depression, or euphoria. Also any candida yeast infections may flare up.

A person who has been on steroids for more than a few weeks must not suddenly stop them, because there may be suppression of their adrenal cortical glands or even shrinking, and then dangerously low blood levels of cortisone result. If long-term treatment is to be stopped, the dose has to be lowered very gradually over a period of time, and under medical supervision.

There *are* conditions where steroids save lives, and also of course if the adrenal or pituitary glands are diseased or damaged, then life-long replacement steroid therapy is essential. However, steroids are *not* recommended in ME, and the side effects strongly outweigh any short-term suppression of symptoms.

Oral contraceptives

'The pill' was hailed as the answer to contraception difficulties and overpopulation in many countries. However certain long-term problems from its use have become recognized. Female hormones are related to cortisone in their chemical structure, and artificially high levels induced by synthetic hormone-like chemicals can have some of the effects of steroids – weight gain, mental changes, and candida yeast overgrowth.

Oral contraceptives also lead to depletion of zinc, and raised copper levels. There is increased tendency to allergies, migraines, blood clotting, high blood pressure and depression. Some of the mental symptoms may be due to the disturbance of B vitamin metabolism by the pill, particularly B_1, B_6 and B_{12}, and to the low zinc/high copper change.

So it is evident that women with ME, who may have enough problems with depression, thrush, sugar metabolism and vitamin and mineral malabsorption, should *not* create further problems by taking the pill.

There is evidence to show that long-term effects of being on the pill for several years include increased susceptibility to allergies, and less resistance to infections, indicating some changes in immune response.

Anaesthetics and surgery

All anaesthetic agents are drugs with powerful effects on the central nervous system. Any after effects are likely to be much more severe for an ME sufferer, and there may be increased risk of liver damage by inhalation agents such as Halothane. I know of two cases where the effect of a muscle paralysing drug (routinely used in anaesthesia after you have gone to sleep to allow a tube to be safely passed down the airway) has taken an abnormally long time to wear off after the operation. Since there appears to be some disturbance of neuro-transmitters between nerve cells, and also some disturbance of muscle function in ME, it is not surprising that a routine anaesthetic may cause problems. Obviously there may be occasions when surgery is absolutely essential; you would not wish to delay operating on acute appendicitis, or a badly broken leg!

If surgery is really needed, it is important that you tell the anaesthetist you have ME, and describe any problems you may have with muscles, walking, co-ordination and brain symptoms. Then he or she can make adjustments and use the most appropriate drugs in lower doses if necessary.

Of course, any operation and any anaesthetic is highly stressful, and is very likely to bring on some relapse. If it is unavoidable, then try to make provision for extra care and rest in the convalescent period and take extra vitamin C, zinc, vitamin A and all B vitamins for a few weeks after surgery. Allow yourself plenty of time to recover.

Otherwise, if you have to make some decision about whether to go on a waiting list for non-urgent surgery – e.g. varicose veins, hysterectomy, bunionectomy, lumpectomies, etc., it is always possible that if you have ME and try to change your life to have rest, less stress, and better nutrition, there may follow some improvement in the condition for which you were going to have an operation. This would apply especially to abnormal bleeding, for which a lot of women end up having possibly unnecessary hysterectomies. Any non-essential orthopaedic procedures should be postponed until the ME is better.

Pregnancy and Labour

The question of drugs, such as pain killers, gas and air, epidurals, etc., for women in childbirth, is one to discuss beforehand with the obstetrician and midwife. Many women with ME do cope quite well with pregnancy and labour, and it is common sense to let the health workers concerned with the pregnancy and delivery know in advance about the ME.

Pregnancy seems to make ME better for some women. However the worst problems come once the new baby is at home, and there is the inevitable lack of sleep, exhaustion and post-natal blues which are all going to seem worse in someone with ME. A relapse at this time may be inevitable.

However, the joy of a new child may well outweigh the problems, and decisions about embarking on a pregnancy are so individual, that it is quite out of place to give pro or con advice in this book.

There is no way that ME harms an unborn baby, nor has it ever been reported that a mother passed on ME to a small child. So there is no medical reason for not having a baby, except for the problems of how an ill and exhausted mother can cope with a small child. Some women seem to have started their ME after a pregnancy.

Local Anaesthetic

Many ME sufferers report increased sensitivity to local anaesthetic. It may be an over-reaction to the adrenaline which is often combined with the anaesthetic, and it is wise to ask the dental surgeon to use local anaesthetic without adrenaline. Several instances of ME sufferers collapsing or losing consciousness after local anaesthesia for dental procedures have been recorded. On the other hand, many muscle biopsies have been performed on ME patients, with no ill effect from the local anaesthetic. So the reactions experienced in the dentist's chair may be partly due to stress from dentist phobia, or to the site of injection being more closely related to cranial structures, or to the dose used.

Whatever the reasons, non-urgent dental treatment, apart from scaling and cleaning, is probably not a good idea while you are unwell with ME. Candida often lurks in the mouth and in gum crevices, so good preventative mouth and gum hygiene is extremely important. You may find that the health of your gums improves after cutting out sugar and eating a lot more vegetables, and increasing vitamin C intake.

Mercury Toxicity – is it Relevant?

Talking of dental treatment, another reason why some ME patients report a relapse following dental work involving fillings may be to do with mercury sensitivity. Now this is a highly controversial topic, and whole books have been written on the subject.

What are the facts?

We know that mercury is extremely poisonous. It is used in a mixture with silver, tin, copper and zinc, containing about 50 per cent mercury. Once the amalgam has been installed in the tooth, there is no proof that some of the mercury does not escape in the form of vapour and enter the body. When the fillings are ground as in chewing, some mercury *does* escape as vapour, this can enter the saliva and be swallowed, and can be converted into methyl mercury by the action of bacteria in the mouth and in the gut. Methyl mercury is much more toxic than elemental mercury.

Because there is more than one metal in the mouth and there is liquid in the form of saliva, a small but measurable electric current is continuously generated in the mouth. This is one thing that gradually corrodes the amalgam, together with foodstuffs and chemicals, and physical wearing away by chewing. All amalgam fillings gradually deteriorate, some have to be replaced after five to ten years. So where has the mercury gone?

The electric potentials between teeth and their surrounding saliva can be measured using a milliammeter. Some of the symptoms which may be due to the electric current in the mouth, which has been measured as 900 mv or more, include:

> Metallic taste in the mouth, increased salivation, irritability, pins and needles or pain in the face, and severe depression. The roots of teeth, particularly in the upper jaw, pass close to main nerves, and the impulses passing along nerves can be affected by local electric currents. So it is not implausible that a variety of head symptoms, such as pain, 'tics', visual problems, disturbances in taste and other sensations, might be resulting from the presence of electric potentials in the mouth.

Research has demonstrated that mercury can affect central nervous system functioning, and also has a bad effect on the immune system. It was demonstrated in 1984 that removal of amalgam fillings resulted in a rise in circulating T lymphocytes, whose numbers fell when the amalgam was reinserted. This may be due to hypersensitivity to amalgam fillings. There is certainly plenty of documented evidence of the undesirable results of having such a toxic metal in the mouth. However, at the present time, I believe that the majority of dental surgeons in the UK still maintain that mercury amalgam fillings are quite safe, and that there are no long-term health hazards.

For those readers who would like to pursue this matter further, I recommend the book *The Toxic Time Bomb*, by Sam Ziff.

Now the problem for someone whose illness has been diagnosed as ME, and who has rows of old standard amalgam fillings, is this. Do you rush off and ask your dentist to take them all out and replace them with one of the newer metal-free fillings?

There are several snags about this:

- The replacement is not available on the NHS and will therefore be costly in the UK.
- You need to have evidence first that the amalgam is causing trouble, which is hard to find. However, it is possible to have tests done which show if the mercury is leaking out, and if you are allergic to it. These tests are only available from a few dentists.
- The process of removing amalgam causes a great release of mercury, and usually the patient feels much worse for some days, maybe longer. In other words, it may induce a severe relapse.
- The removal needs to be done by a dentist who is aware of the hazards, with special precautions taken to minimize swallowing and inhaling amalgam. The fillings need to be removed in a particular sequence, depending on which ones are causing the greatest reaction.
- Some of the replacement materials may cause problems. Ideally the patient needs to be tested for sensitivity to different substitute materials beforehand.
- Because it is a procedure which causes extra stress and worsening of symptoms, it is essential to take extra supplements of vitamins C, B complex, A, pantothenic acid and zinc before and for several weeks afterwards.

There is an urgent need for more research into the connections between mercury amalgam fillings and immune functioning, hormone production, the nervous system and, indeed, the whole physiology of the body. Some figures on ME sufferers and healthy controls are needed, to see if the percentage of those with amalgam fillings is significantly different from the percentage of non-ME population with amalgam. At the present time, nobody really knows.

Mercury toxicity is one of a number of environmental factors to be considered when studying ME and its causes.

In the meantime, the advice to ME patients about changing dental fillings is this. **Do not rush off and have amalgam removed**, especially if you are really ill. If you start to get better, and feel you would like advice about it, contact the British Dental Society for Clinical Nutrition (address in Appendix A).

Immunizations

An immunization is a procedure in which the body's immune system is stimulated to produce an antibody to a specific infection; so that if the virus or bacteria causing the infection enters the body at a later date, the white blood cells will recognize it and produce lots more antibody very quickly. The antigen, or stimulus for making antibody, is usually a form of virus or bacteria which has been killed, or changed so as to make it harmless (this latter is called 'live attenuated virus' vaccine). When smallpox immunization was given, a modified relative called cowpox was used.

The question of immunization for an ME sufferer is only likely to arise in two circumstances.

(a) before foreign travel – e.g. typhoid, cholera, yellow-fever prevention, or polio booster;
(b) to start or boost protection against tetanus, for going abroad, for gardeners and agricultural or forest workers, or when there is a penetrating wound.

Practically all ME sufferers will have had the usual childhood 'jabs', i.e. tetanus, diptheria, polio, small-pox, BCG (for TB), possibly measles. I have not yet discovered any ME person who actually knows he or she has had *no* immunizations at all.

If tetanus protection is advised, this should be done, because tetanus toxoid does not involve the injection of actual bacteria, but of a derivative of the tetanus toxin, and has no record of bad effects. Full blown tetanus disease is lethal, and no one should need to die from it.

So the main occasion when you may query having an immunization is before going abroad. Unless it is obligatory before entering the foreign country, the advice to ME patients is **don't have immunizations**.

Typhoid and cholera (commonly given together as TAB/cho) jabs cause some reaction in all healthy people, and may lead to a severe reaction, a relapse, or possibly to *no* reaction at all, in someone with ME. The lack of any reaction may mean that no immunity develops, and the person eats and drinks contaminated food in the belief that he or she is protected.

It is better not to go to countries with high risk of enteric diseases; if you go, though, be scrupulously careful about hygiene, boiling water, and not eating uncooked food in cafés, etc. Anyway, typhoid and cholera injections do not protect against dysentery and hepatitis, which are just as easily picked up in many countries.

So the general advice about immunizations and ME is to avoid them, unless it is tetanus toxoid. Immunizations are intended to stir up the immune system, but if the immune system is not functioning quite normally, one can end up with hypersensitivity reactions, or incomplete immunity.

There is no evidence at present which links earlier immunizations with diseases such as ME. However, an article in the *Lancet* (January 1985) mentioned research in Europe which demonstrated measles virus particles in the bodies of adults with chronic illness.

We know that in ME the virus exists in cells and alters their function. Immunization is another factor in the history of ME sufferers which needs to be investigated.

Some Useful Drugs

Ideally, it would be best to do without any medicines at all. The main emphasis with ME should be on rest, good nutrition, and natural ways of removing stresses to the immune system and allowing the body to heal itself.

However there may be occasions when certain medicines can help tide one over a bad patch, and assist in dealing with troublesome symptoms. The important thing is not to view the medicine as getting you better on its own. It is just a prop, and should be discarded when no longer needed, or if it causes more symptoms than it is treating.

As you have probably found out, much of living with ME turns out to be compromise. There are sensible rules to follow, which can sometimes be broken. The rigidly obsessive personality whose life is dominated by strict rules is not going to be relaxed enough to get better.

Sleeping Pills – if these really are needed and other measures don't help, then one of the gentle short-acting hypnotics is best, such as Temazepam or Triazolam, starting with a small dose.

Sedatives – if there is extreme anxiety and agitation with insomnia, then a very small dose of a drug such as Thioridazine 30 mg at night has been found helpful for short periods by some patients.

Antihistamines – Piriton, in small doses such as 2 to 4 mg twice daily, can be very helpful if there are many allergic symptoms, particularly the chronic explosive sneezing and streaming nose experienced by some sufferers. It causes a little sedation, but if taken at night, this is no disadvantage.

Nalcrom (sodium cromoglycate) – this may be helpful to prevent reactions in severely food allergic patients, if they are in a situation where they cannot control their diet. One or two 100 mg capsules are taken before meals, either whole, or contents dissolved in water (see page 164).

Painkillers – avoid aspirin, and compounds containing aspirin. Many people are sensitive to salycilates, and aspirin is now known to cause allergic responses and may be implicated in a hypersensitivity illness in children called Reye's syndrome. It is also irritant on the stomach. All the non-steroid anti-inflammatory drugs have the potential for gastric irritation, ulcers and hypersensitivity reactions.

Ipobrufen (Brufen) is an anti-inflammatory drug that

can be used for headaches, joint pain and period pain, in low dose.

Paracetamol has fewer side effects than aspirin; again a small dose should be tried, such as 1/2 tablet instead of two tablets.

A good remedy for pain is vitamin C, a gram every hour. It has anti-prostaglandin effects similar to aspirin and anti-inflammatory drugs, and is much safer!

Treatment for Constipation

Changes in bowel habit are very common with ME. Sometimes constipation and diarrhoea alternate. Constipation should be avoided, as it leads to greater chance of absorption of toxins from the large bowel, and more fermentation of any undigested food which reaches the colon. It may result in bad smelling wind, and abdominal discomfort. Some people pass a bowel motion only once every two days; for them this may be normal. The more usual pattern in health is to defaecate between one and three times a day. The bulk produced is greater when the diet is very high in vegetables and wholegrains.

The best way to deal with constipation, or if you feel you need a clearout, is to drink plenty of water between meals, take extra vitamin C, several grams as necessary, plus extra magnesium, maybe 200 mg or so, or Milk of Magnesia, or a dose of liver salts on occasions. If you really need a laxative other than vitamin C and magnesium, stick to those based on plants, such as syrup of figs or sennokot, and still take plenty of water with them. Glycerin suppositories can be used sometimes with no harmful effects. Linusit (from linseeds) and sesame seeds are very helpful for constipation.

Improving the balance of good bugs in the colon, such as taking Probion, drinking plenty of fluids, and having masses of fibre from vegetables and fruit are the key to dealing with chronic constipation.

Anti-depressants

These do seem to be very useful for ME symptoms apart from depression in some patients, although may not influence the time taken for complete recovery. (See the section on anti-depressants in the chapter on depression, page 213.)

Case History

The following history is of someone whose ME syndrome seemed to be triggered by dental treatment.

MR A. G. AGE AT ONSET 54 EX-TEACHER (NOW CHIROPODIST)

In 1965, following dentistry and amalgam fillings, I suffered very bad trembling, exhaustion and loss of oxygen. I was subjected to tests in hospital, all were negative. I went home, but could not walk for six weeks. I resumed my life with difficulty at first, then gradually recovered.

In 1985, I had an abscess on a tooth, and went to a dentist. Five amalgam fillings. I returned home in August feeling hot, weak and ill and was sent to hospital with suspected thrombosis. A large black bruise appeared on my leg. All tests were negative, although I was regarded as a 'cheat' and was shouted at by the consultant, who said I *could walk*. Back home, again unable to cross a room for weeks.

My wife, who is interested in natural medicine,

got me moving with calcium pantothenate prolonged release capsules. I was also treated by a London homeopath who advised potassium, which helped.

Since then, my symptoms have been: inability to walk sometimes, shortness of breath, pain in the left side and in legs, distortion of vision and hearing, and dizziness. All symptoms come and go with periods of remission and relapse.

I am now doing very well, thanks to vitamins in supplementary liquid form, and thanks always to homeopathy and herbs. I was no 'health crank' or 'faddist', I may say. I was simply driven to use these methods of healing when the orthodox failed me. That failing of the formal orthodox was very traumatic, but I did learn the true and incomparable value of these older medicines.

I have some remaining damage, I may say, to my nervous system. *This* recovery may be slow. I also have a very curious reaction: I overheat after eating, but especially after hot/warm drinks. I have a deep seated 'sugar imbalance' also. Yet I do not have diabetes: perhaps the opposite? I have a dread of tooth decay, not without cause. Having some perhaps temporary damage to my immune system, as it appeared, and requiring tooth extraction (the only way to get rid of mercury amalgam at that time), I reacted badly and suffered severe mouth infection. I then resorted to Ferr. Phos. which stopped the mouth decay over two weeks of terrible fear.

My feeling is that ME is a 'surface condition', and that another something lies beneath. For myself, as perhaps for others, I feel that the key is *hypoglycaemia*. It is only now, in my fifties, that I am able to look back and see a pattern to my health life. I was unnaturally hungry as a child. I was passed Grade I RAF Nat. Service in 1951, and I was also a medallist racing cyclist as well as a cricketer. And yet I suffered occasional 'black-outs' or 'faints'. I also had to eat regularly.

I wonder if many others are hypoglycaemic and do not know it? I suffer many of the symptoms of a diabetic, and have lived on a 'home-made' diet for 15 years. I have given up potatoes, white bread, and have brown bread and brown rice. I have to have meat for strength. I also need a little salt. Sometimes glucose will remove the pain in my side.

I think (my own theory) that the mercury threw my metabolic body out of gear.

Suggested Further Reading

The Toxic Time Bomb, by Sam Ziff (Thorsons, 1984).
The Bitter Pill, by Dr Ellen Grant (Elm Tree Books, 1985).

17

Homeopathy and Other Therapies

If you suffer from an illness which goes on and on, for which conventional medicine has no answers, it is likely that you will look for help from the traditional forms of healing. The art of healing is as old as mankind, and all ways of healing have this common purpose.

To heal is to make whole, and healing means restoring wholeness. The word health comes from the word 'hale', meaning whole, hence the term (w)holistic medicine. Lack of health implies disintegration, loss of balance, disorder of the fine tuning of mental, spiritual and bodily functions. Symptoms are messages that things are not flowing smoothly within us. Many drugs just suppress these important messages, whereas most non-drug therapies seek to correct the underlying imbalance by helping the body to restore its own wholeness.

There is of course a lot of overlap between modern Western medicine and the so called 'alternative' therapies. The visit to a doctor who also has a gift for healing (which is not given to all, in spite of degrees, diplomas, and modern technology), is in itself therapeutic.

You tell your complete story to someone who is prepared to listen. You receive words of explanation and comfort, and the touch of healing hands through a handshake or examination. You may be given a prescription for a medicine, and *you are encouraged to believe that it will help you.*

The patient's belief that something will do good is an important part of any therapy, whether it is a bottle of painkillers, of stomach medicine, or homeopathic remedies, acupuncture, manipulation or whatever. This is sometimes called the *placebo effect*, and is a universal natural part of healing. It is perfectly valid in all forms of healing, whether the healer is a witch-doctor, an eminent Harley Street specialist, a family doctor, a professor or a herbalist.

The mind and the body cannot be separated; diseases that originate from a psychological disorder may show up as physical symptoms; those that have a purely physical cause may initially present with psychological symptoms. ME is a condition whose origin may be a virus, but the patient is very depressed. Its initial cause may be prolonged mental stress, but the main symptom can be muscle pain.

Does it matter if a condition of ill health is classified as 'organic' or as 'psychological'? I think it does not, and indeed to try to argue for one or the other is futile in a condition such as ME, because with each individual sufferer one is looking at a body-mind-spirit complex which is disordered, and would like to be whole again.

So the patient's belief in the possibility of improvement is quite a significant part of any healing therapy. This is due to the influence that mental attitude has over bodily recovery. It is known that among people with a serious illness such as cancer, those who have an optimistic outlook with a reason for staying alive do better than those who are pessimists with feelings of helplessness.

ME sufferers who get better report a great range of reasons for their recovery. Some say that homeopathy cured them, some benefit from exclusion diets and treating candida, some have improved after the laying on of hands in Christian healing; virtually all say they needed to rest to get better.

It cannot be repeated too often that *you need to rest, whatever else you undertake in the search for healing*! The energy expenditure involved in travelling up and down the country, looking for a therapist who will cure you, may undo the benefits of therapy, depending on how many visits are needed and how well you stand up to travelling.

Homeopathy

The word 'homeopathy' comes from two Greek words, *homois* and *pathos* meaning *similar* and *suffering*.

A homeopathic remedy is one which produces similar symptoms to those of the patient, when taken in its undiluted form by a healthy person. Homeopathy follows the principle of 'like treats like', unlike allopathic Western medicine which treats symptoms by substances with opposite effects.

An example of homeopathic medicine which was actually used as a conventional drug is quinine. This is derived from the bark of a tree, which if taken over some time produces symptoms of shivering, sweating and fever. A weaker extract of this tree bark is prepared as the drug quinine and was used to treat malaria.

A homeopathic remedy is prepared by diluting the medicine many times, in a process of serial dilutions called 'potentization'. In the resulting dilution, there may be few or no molecules of the original substance left; however during the dilution process the mixture is shaken very vigorously at each stage, and it is thought that some biologically active property of the molecules of the original drug is imparted to the resulting potentized remedy, whether the dilution is with a liquid or a solid.

The weaker the concentration of a remedy, the more highly potentized it is, and the more powerful it is in terms of biological effect. The curative effect would seem to be from a gentle stimulation of the body to put right the imbalance which is causing the symptoms.

A homeopathic remedy is selected after careful history taking to establish not only all the patient's symptoms, but other characteristics such as personality, seasonal influence, food likes and dislikes, factors which influence symptoms, etc. So there is no one remedy which is always prescribed for any one symptom; three patients with rheumatism may each require a different remedy, according to the total symptom and character picture of each patient.

Good homeopathic prescribing requires skill and experience, and it is best to consult a fully trained practitioner. Homeopathy is safe and does not harm the body.

However, when treating a chronic deep-seated condition, it is common to have temporary worsening of symptoms to start with. Some remedies are used to treat symptoms only, and can be bought and self-prescribed for first aid and home use. These are lower potencies, and are very useful for first aid treatment of such things as headache, fever, stomach upsets, bruises, etc. An example of such a remedy is Arnica 6× (meaning diluted 1 in 10 six times), a remedy for bruising, sprains and muscle pain from over-use.

To treat a chronic condition, a higher potency may be used, and fewer doses are taken. The deepest level of homeopathic treatment for ME is given by identifying the infection which is persisting in the body and causing symptoms, then giving a homeopathic preparation of the virus, or whatever germ.

This type of remedy is called a '*nosode*'. Nosodes of other chronic infections, thought to be the long past origins of ill health, have been used in homeopathy for a long time. An example of a classical nosode is tuberculinum, reflecting on how large a part TB used to play in chronic ill health.

The virus nosode used to treat ME is not always of the exact virus, but may be of its family – herpes virus nosode would be suitable for patients whose ill health is related to past glandular fever (Epstein Barr virus), chickenpox, or any other herpes viruses. It is possible to make a homeopathic preparation of any virus, or of whatever is thought to have started off the ME.

There are two difficulties about this homeopathic approach to ME. The first is that of knowing what is the infection which needs to be treated. The homeopathic practitioner may decide on evidence of history – 'I've never been well since glandular fever, chickenpox', or whatever; or on evidence of blood test reports, if these are available, and if they reveal any organism.

Another method of identifying the infectious agent is by sensitivity testing, using the muscle weakness or the Vega test (see page 161), and testing for reactions to bottles containing preparations or extracts of various infections. Candida yeast sensitivity can also be tested for by this method, and indeed a persistent candida overgrowth can be attacked by prescribing homeopathic Candida 30×, which stimulates the body's defences to get rid of it.

The second difficulty is that if the correct nosode is taken, it is likely to induce a temporary revival of all the original symptoms of the infection that triggered off the ME syndrome. This can be hard to bear for a sufferer who had perhaps started a gradual recovery. However, the apparent severe relapse should not last very long, a few days to a few weeks, and should be seen as a *good thing*, a sign that the body is being stirred up to get rid of the persisting infection.

Because of this 'worse before you get better' effect, a careful practitioner tries to help strengthen the patient before using the nosode; by supportive measures, such as improving mineral and vitamin levels, removing major allergies from the diet, and treating candida; and generally strengthening those parts of the body which seem especially stressed, such as the liver, pancreas, kidneys or heart, by using appropriate remedies and advice.

Some remedies that have been mentioned by various ME patients include:

- *Aconite* – for great fear and anxiety, especially at night, for the 'feeling of dying', with pressure on the chest, breathing difficulty, or fluttering heart.
- *Lactic acid* in potency – for muscle pains and ill feeling after any exercise.
- *Arnica* – for aching muscles and joints, exhaustion from overdoing things.
- *Candida* nosode – for candida overgrowth, in combination with other anti-candida measures.
- *Homeopathic interferon* – this has been used on some patients at one alternative medicine centre, apparently with good results.

For further information and advice about the value of homeopathy, you are advised to read one of several excellent books available, or to consult a qualified practitioner.

Celloid Mineral Therapy

Celloid minerals are based on tissue salt therapy devised by Dr Schussler of Germany. The treatment aims to correct mineral deficiencies within living cells which result in illness, or complicate diseases. The actual minerals used in tissue salt and celloid mineral therapy are only those which occur naturally in our bodies and in foods. The minerals are 'potentized' in a similar way to homeopathic remedies; this renders them biologically much more active, at a lower dose per tablet, than would otherwise be needed by taking a straightforward mineral preparation.

Celloid minerals can be taken at the same time as other medication. There are no side effects; however during the early days of taking them, there may be a temporary worsening of symptoms as the chemistry in the body adjusts.

The choice of one or a combination of minerals to prescribe is based on careful history and assessment by a practitioner who has had special training in the principles and use of celloid therapy.

Acupuncture

Many people think of acupuncture as being mainly a treatment for pain. This healing art has been used by the Chinese for thousands of years, and used not only to treat pain, but all kinds of illness, and also to prevent disease from developing.

A Chinese physician does not make diagnoses in the same way as a Western doctor does. In Chinese medicine, a history and examination are carried out but with particular attention to the appearance of the face and tongue, and the quality of the pulse at both wrists. The practitioner is looking for signs of imbalance of body energies, and how the body functions are disturbed.

There is no such diagnosis as ME in Chinese medicine. A patient who presents with complaints of exhaustion, muscle weakness, feeling cold and insomnia, might be regarded as suffering from deficient Yang Chi (*chi* is energy), and deficiency of chi of various organs such as heart, spleen and liver. Another patient may have a slightly different diagnosis, but all ME sufferers are basically lacking in body energy (chi); this is reflected in poor function of organs, cold, stagnation of energy in energy pathways leading to pain, poor digestion and absorption of food, or disturbed mental function.

Acupuncture treatment for ME needs to be given in a way that does not drain energy from the patient, but rather supplies energy, or else stimulates the body's immune system. A technique which supplies energy is to use a burning herb (moxa) over acupuncture-points, the warmth entering the energy channels and dispersing cold and invigorating body organs. The smouldering moxa does not burn the skin, only creates a sensation of heat.

There are also techniques which stimulate the body's production of endorphins – these are natural hormones of well-being and pain relief – and boost the immune system.

There is no single prescription of acupuncture or moxa especially to treat ME, as each patient is assessed individually and a diagnosis is formulated according to one of several systems, which vary in different teaching schedules.

This is mentioned because a patient may consult more than one acupuncturist and find that each uses a different system for making a diagnosis – one may place more emphasis on pulse examination, the other may give greater weight to diagnosis from looking at the tongue.

The hows and whys of an acupuncturist's diagnosis are not important to the patient. What is much more important is to consult a fully trained practitioner, rather than someone who just sticks needles in to relieve pain. The reason for this is that an unskilled acupuncturist may make an ME patient worse, by giving treatment in a way that results in energy being drained away.

Many conditions have painful spots which are treated by draining energy from local areas. If the patient's underlying energy level is normal, i.e. he or she does not have ME, this treatment is fine. But for ME, acupuncture treatment needs to be gentle, and to be given in a way that does *not* remove energy. Most ME patients are extremely sensitive, and may have a greater reaction to acupuncture than other patients.

The insertion of an acupuncture needle is swift and virtually painless. If the needle is then manipulated there is a sensation which varies from a deep ache to a tingling or a numbness – this indicates that the point has been correctly located and the needle will do its work. Few patients complain of pain from acupuncture therapy, and if any is felt, it is short-lived.

On the whole, acupuncture needling is not appropriate for someone in a severe stage of ME, nor for patients who are very sensitive with a lot of muscle pain. Moxa (heat) treatment is more acceptable in such cases. Acupuncture can be very helpful for insomnia, temperature instability, anxiety and some nervous symptoms. I have not come across anyone whose muscle weakness and pain has been significantly improved, and rest and good nutrition should still be prescribed in addition to acupuncture.

Massage and Aromatherapy

Many sufferers seem to find massage helpful. If you cannot find a trained therapist locally, or cannot go out for treatment, it may be worth finding a book which describes simple massage techniques for a carer to learn.

The massage needs to be extremely gentle, especially if the sufferer is very ill or has a lot of body pain. There is no place for the vigorous pummelling and rubbing endured by James Bond-like characters in steaming Turkish baths!

Many of the benefits of massage come from the physical touch of a caring person, just as a mother soothes a child by stroking its head. The emphasis should be on comforting, soothing and relaxing rather than on trying to massage away muscle pain. The body is so sensitive in ME, that a much lighter touch is needed than in massage for a fit person.

Aromatherapy is performed by a practitioner who is trained in massage, and also uses essential oils on the skin for their therapeutic properties rather than just a skin lubricant. After an initial consultation, an aromatherapist may give you a supply of the oils he or she has used, for you to rub in yourself at home, or add a few drops to the bath. The prescription used will be individual to your needs, based on the chief symptoms. The oils are very pure extracts from various plants which have healing properties known for centuries. They do not contain colourings or chemicals; minute amounts are absorbed through the skin, and fragrance is inhaled, to produce their beneficial effects.

Essential oils work on one level by relieving stress and anxiety, and at a deeper level they can balance body energies and benefit the immune system. Different oils are used for different emotional and physical problems; some have stimulating properties (such as eucalyptus), others affect functions like digestion and hormone levels.

Oils with stimulating properties should not be used on people with ME.

Those who have tried aromatherapy have found it very pleasant and comforting. Benefits include muscle relaxation, less muscle pain, better sleep and less anxiety. If a practitioner can be found who can visit at home, so much the better.

Reflexology

Reflexology works on reflex points of the body, mainly on the feet; the points have connections to specific body areas. The connections are thought to be either via nerve endings, or via channels of energy. A reflexology therapist may find that reflex points, which correspond to areas of the body causing symptoms, are congested and tender. Pressing and massaging points on the sole of a foot can balance body energies, and stimulate glands and organs to function better.

There are connections between the practice of reflexology and ancient Chinese acupressure, where the principles are the same as in acupuncture but the points are stimulated by finger pressure instead of needles.

Reflex points in other areas of the body can be used, although those of feet and hands are the main ones. Even simple massage of the feet is very relaxing and also toning to the body. Those ME sufferers who have tried reflexology have reported that it is pleasant, helps many symptoms, and has no harmful effects.

Yoga

This is not strictly regarded as a therapy, however yoga has great benefits for circulation, breathing, and seems to improve blood flow to the extremities and hence oxygenation of tissues.

However, yoga is only suitable for ME sufferers who are relatively well, and the inverted postures which place strain on the neck must be avoided, as must any posture which needs prolonged muscle tension to maintain it. The yoga teacher should be told if you have ME, and you should not push yourself in any way. The most useful aspect of yoga, the breathing and calmness, can be carried out at home, even sitting in a chair.

T'ai Chi chu'an

T'ai Chi is a very ancient, gentle, martial art, performed as a traditional series of movements that are intended to unite body and mind. It was developed many centuries ago, and is widely practised in China, Japan, and other countries round the world, for health, meditation, and self-defence and enjoyment.

You may be astonished to read that 'a martial art' is described in a self-help book for ME sufferers! But the movements in T'ai Chi are very gentle and flowing, more like a dance, no force or sudden muscular effort is used at all. It can be learnt by people of any age, weak or strong. Each muscle changes very gently between use and relaxation; there is improvement of muscle tone, of circulation of blood and lymphatics, there is gentle movement of all joints, and the slow turning of the body massages internal organs. There is calming of mind and body, and deep regular breathing.

There is on record that a T'ai Chi master, T. T. Liang, learned the art in middle age, after many operations and prolonged illness. He not only confounded doctors who had predicted imminent death, but practised it at the age of 77 to preserve his health.

Now there may be many ME sufferers who are not well enough to learn T'ai Chi, because it is performed standing up, and taking slow steps and paces and moving the arms, which may be too weak to be held up. It is recommended for sufferers who are getting better or are in remission, especially those whose muscle weakness or pain is not so severe. Once learnt, T'ai Chi can be performed at home as well as in a class. Even doing a few movements for a few minutes between spells of lying down can be beneficial.

Bach Flower Remedies

Bach Remedies are made from various different plants, each of which has a specific effect on a disordered emotional state. They are different from herbal preparations, in that they are very dilute pure preparations and work exclusively on the emotions rather than on other bodily symptoms. They are absolutely safe, and if a remedy is chosen which is inappropriate for the emotional state, there is no harmful effect.

The most useful to keep at hand is Bach's Rescue Remedy, which is made from five specific remedies, and is used in a situation of sudden mental shock or collapse. Another useful remedy is Olive, which helps a fatigued exhausted mind.

Herbal Medicine

Plants with specific healing properties have been used to prepare medicines, poultices, powders, etc., for a very long time, throughout the world. Some of our modern drugs are derived from plant medicines, for example Digoxin, used for heart failure, is a purified product of the leaves of digitalis, the foxglove.

On the whole, herbal medicines are safer than modern synthetic drugs, so long as they are taken in the prescribed way. A qualified medical herbalist does several years of training, that includes anatomy and physiology and study of illness (pathology), as well as learning a vast amount of botany and pharmacology of plants. For first aid use at home, herbal remedies are available from herbalists, many pharmacists and at health food shops, and these medicines are all quite safe.

For treatment of chronic ailments and deep-seated symptoms, it is best to consult a qualified herbalist. He or she will take a detailed history, and will prescribe a herb, or more usually, a combination of herbs, not just to suppress symptoms, but to help correct the cause of illness. Chinese medicine actually uses herbs as much as acupuncture, more in China itself, and there are many similarities in the mode of diagnosis and prescription between Chinese herbal medicine, and herbal medicine as taught in Western countries.

The property of a plant for healing purposes is not classified as being 'good for cough' (for example), but rather in terms of its functions of heating or cooling, stimulating or sedating, contracting or relaxing of smooth muscle, antiseptic, blood purifying, etc. Some are particularly rich in essential minerals which may be depleted in disease.

Some of the commonest herbs are found in our

gardens and kitchens, such as onion, garlic, parsley, thyme, mint, sage, ginger, cayenne. Many familiar garden plants have powerful properties, including nettles, dandelions and marigold.

Many herbal preparations have side effects *if used incorrectly* or if the wrong part of a plant is used, but the toxic side effects are not as common as occur from use of synthetic chemical drugs.

There are certain herbs that have anti-viral properties. One of these is Hydrastis Canadensis – commonly known as golden seal. Another is Allium Sativum – which is garlic, and is well known as an anti-infection plant.

Herbal teas are good as alternatives to tea or coffee. There are a good variety available now. It is helpful to know their different properties – for example peppermint aids digestion, and chamomile is a natural sedative and suitable for the evening.

There are of course many other therapies which have not been mentioned here; this is not because they are unknown or useless. Those described in this chapter have all been helpful to some ME sufferers. It appears that homeopathy has helped more people than others; but in the absence of any organized trial of different therapies, for a 'standardized' group of ME patients, any evidence of one treatment being better than another is anecdotal.

Case History

The following case history describes the use of Chinese herbalism.

MR F. L. AGE AT ONSET 52 OCCUPATION – UNIVERSITY LECTURER

September 1985 – My illness started suddenly with acute gastro-enteritis while in Zimbabwe. I was treated with a broad spectrum antibiotic (chloramphenicol). Shortly after, I returned to England. Two weeks later, I felt more ill, weak physically, and the tongue became very sore and shed its surface. Given nystatin suspension. Blood and stool specimens examined, nothing abnormal found.

October 1985 – Gradually recovered strength, got back to normal life and teaching, but over the winter and spring I had periods of feeling very tired and weak, had more sore throats than usual.

April 1986 – As a preliminary to dental treatment, commenced a course of broad spectrum antibiotic (Amoxyl). Following this, I found I was becoming quite ill after each weekend of physical activity, the fatigue lasting four days. My tongue became thickly coated.

June 1986 – I sought medical advice. I had a thorough check up with numerous tests, nothing abnormal found. Meanwhile there were times when I was very ill indeed:

> physically weak, overtired, headaches; very sore throat and earache; sore mouth and lips; frequent light-headedness, and at times I could not co-ordinate my speech. I often woke up with tingling in the muscles and headache.

I was given the diagnosis of 'post viral fatigue', but was not given any advice about rest. The hospital consultant wanted to prescribe anti-depressants for my emotional lability, which I refused to take.

I then tried the anti-candida diet, and a course of nystatin, with no improvement. Homeopathic testing, and a swab of mouth ulcers, revealed no candida.

It probably took about 12 months to accept that a cure could not be effected quickly, and that full recovery would be a protracted business. I formed the opinion that a 'holistic approach' is the only effective strategy for dealing with the problem, and that this must involve both the body and the mind. Being very much a pragmatic person, I decided at a very early stage that I must tackle my situation in a practical, business-like manner. This has meant that I have adjusted my tactics over the years to suit changes in my condition and circumstances.

I seem to have two main problems:

(1) malfunction of my muscles (and, when very ill, of my nervous system);
(2) malfunction of my lower intestine. If anything, malfunction of the intestine often seems to exert the dominant effect. For example, before I became ill, my stools were always formed and I had tendencies towards constipation. Since becoming ill, the opposite applies; my stools are only formed when I am feeling really well ('pseudo-recovery'), which has only happened on a few occasions over the last three years. This particularly interests me, because medical interest always seems to ignore the bowel, even though enteroviruses are often invoked as being a cause of ME. In so far as I am concerned, this was almost certainly the origin of my illness.

For most of the last year, I have adopted two strategies for treatment: I regularly take traditional Chinese herbal medicine (for my body); and have been trying to stabilize my bowel by various means.

The herbal medicine is prescribed by a doctor from mainland China. She was recommended by the Chinese Embassy, and I was introduced to her by my Chinese research student at a time when I was so ill that I could not manage more than one flight of stairs, and I was spending most of the day in bed.

Apart from a lapse of eight months, when I was well for about half that time and ill, with varying degrees of intensity, for the remainder, she has been treating me for most of the three years that I have been affected. I have been very impressed with her approach, and I have no doubts that I owe a great deal to her.

She has restored me to something approaching normality on two occasions now; and there is no doubt that my pulse is stronger and my body warmer than may have even been the case before I became ill. (My blood pressure was always low, and my body temperature always about 1°F below normal.)

The medicine is expensive – about £5 per pack of herbs, it is unpleasant to take, and it is a nuisance to prepare. The herbs have to be cut into small pieces, mixed with about 1.5 l of water and simmered 1–1½ hours until the volume of liquor is about 300 ml. The hot liquor is then strained off and taken immediately. When I was very ill, I was having a pack every day; this has now been reduced to two packs a week.

At present, I visit the Chinese doctor about once every six weeks (when I was ill, it was every two weeks). She changes my prescription to suit my condition, mainly diagnosed by pulse, although the medicine has been essentially the same over the last few months. The formulation is incredibly specific: e.g. increases in the 'warmth of the body'. Perhaps I should add that she is also a registered acupuncturist, and that she is qualified to practise Western medicine in China.

As I have stated above, in my case, I believe gut-involvement to be most important. One of the sad things about my illness is that, when I first became very ill, I repeatedly stated this conviction to the doctors who were trying to diagnose my condition. However, once microbiological examination of my stools revealed nothing pathogenic, my suggestion was totally discounted; and, when I persisted in this point of view, there were hints that I was becoming paranoid.

Subsequently, I have formed the opinion that the various 'allergic manifestations' of my condition are also due to some form of gut-involvement. I would suggest that these effects are due to toxins/allergens that somehow cross the gut wall. In this respect, it is worth noting that the Chinese doctor insists that I drink plenty of warm water, which I endeavour to do (as do many Chinese). This, she says, is to eliminate toxins from the body. That I can usually stop the tingling of my lips by drinking two glasses of water tends to corroborate this.

When I went to see a homeopathist (January 1987), who claimed to be able to diagnose candidal infections of the gut, he said that this was definitely not my problem. I was taking nystatin at the time. Instead, he said that I had an imbalance of the gut flora (dysbiosis). He prescribed drops which I took in water, whilst still continuing with the herbal medicine.

After about two weeks, there was a distinct improvement: my stools started to become normal; the coating on my tongue began to disappear; and I began to feel well. About a month later, I was almost back to normal and even physically active. At this stage (February 1987), I stopped taking the herbal medicine because I felt so well, although I kept taking the homeopathic preparation.

Because of excessive pressure at my work I became ill again in May 1987. In mid-October, I again started on the herbal medicine. Its effects were pretty immediate, and the dose has been progressively reduced since that time.

Unfortunately, the effects of the homeopathic preparation on my bowel were not as beneficial as they were before. About six weeks ago, at morning and night, I started to take a carton (150 ml) of what is essentially Acidophilus Yoghourt. We prepare this ourselves in a domestic yoghourt maker. We use a semi-skimmed UHT milk as the growth medium, and a starter culture prepared from 'Quest' 'Non-Dairy Acidophilus Plus' (contains Lactobacillus acidophilus, L. rhamnosus, L. bifidus, and L. faecium). This approach seems to be very helpful, my stools are gradually becoming more formed, and I am much encouraged.

I have been taking supplementary vitamins for over twenty years. I now take more than ever.

I have now accepted that I may never fully recover, although I earnestly hope that this will not be the case.

To me, it has been important to feel useful and to be interested in something. There are times when I have felt so inadequate and unable to cope that I have been very close to seeking release from my employment on medical grounds. I am glad that I did not do so, although the inclination was very strong.

I would advise anyone contemplating this that it should only be done as a very last resort; and I would also point out that, in any case, such major decisions should never be taken when in poor physical and emotional shape. It is much better to use the income to buy in help, than to lose it altogether. Furthermore, there is bound to be some improvement in the future;

and, when this happens, to be without a job could be disastrous both emotionally and financially.

Suggested Further Reading

Homeopathy – the Family Handbook (Allen & Unwin, 1987).
Aromatherapy for Everyone, by Robert Tisserand (Penguin, 1988).
The Home Herbal, by Barbara Griggs (Pan, 1986).
Yoga Self-Taught, by Andre van Lysebeth (Allen & Unwin, 1988).

18

Practical Problems – Finance, Mobility

It is bad enough to have a disabling disease with pain and exhaustion, but many people with ME endure the added stress of financial hardship, through being unable to work. Many are highly motivated, hard-working, self-reliant people, to whom the idea of accepting state benefit may have been unthinkable before natural retirement.

The specific recommendations and addresses given in the next few pages relate to the UK; addresses which sufferers in other countries may contact are listed in Appendix A. The general principles and advice apply, of course, to everyone.

To begin with, when you are ill, you may be in an employed position, and eligible for sick pay. If you are self-employed, you may be able to get Sickness Benefit if you live in Britain.

The real problems arise when you are still ill after six months (28 weeks), and you and everyone else start to wonder how long this is going to go on for. If you are making some recovery, it may be tempting to try going back to work. If the job is full-time, and physically and emotionally demanding – such as nursing or teaching – the chances are that you quickly find out that you are *not* fully recovered, and have to stop work again, and have a major relapse brought on by the exertion. No one can predict if you will need a further six months off, or a year, or two years . . .

You must accept that *your health comes first*, and if you need more time completely off work, that is what has to happen. Some people may be able to negotiate part-time work, with the flexibility of going home or resting should the energy run out. These kinds of jobs are rare. When considering whether or not to stop work completely, you need to ask yourself if the job is going to hinder further recovery, or if you can manage to improve despite the job.

It may turn out to be possible to work only if a lot of other activities are given up, and with someone looking after your domestic needs – shopping, preparing meals, cleaning and laundry. For some people, getting back to some sort of work, even if part-time, will have positive results in mental well-being, and remove the threats of isolation, uselessness and invalidism.

If there is any doubt about your ability to return to work without having a relapse, think carefully.

I struggled for a few months, doing only one day a week to have a minimum income, and found that it took all week to get over the exhaustion caused by one day of light work. Once I decided to stop completely and make the commitment to getting better, some slow recovery started.

A lot will depend on whether you are self-employed and your own boss, or if employed, on the attitude and sympathy of your employer.

You should also consider whether you can really be effective in your job, before you are well enough. It may turn out that clients, pupils, patients, or colleagues suffer from the days when you are struggling and mentally under par, even though *you* may believe you are doing a tremendous job.

So the message is this:

- Do not be too proud to claim state benefits.

- Do not think your presence at work is vital for the world to go round.
- Remember there are thousands of other hard-working, conscientious – maybe cleverer – people just like you who have had to stop working, you are not unique.

See if there is a way of working part-time, with the flexibility to rest or go home if you feel ill. Access to a couch somewhere at work, to have a sleep mid morning or midday, may enable you to stay in your job.

What if work is unpaid and is essential? I am of course referring to that highly underrated profession called 'housewife'. The reasons for stopping work and resting apply to you as well, but the practicalities are difficult. If you cannot run your home, shop or prepare meals, the Social Services Department may be able to pay for a home help, especially if you live alone or are a single parent. You may be entitled to a home help even if you are supported financially, if your husband or partner has a busy job and is out most of each day.

If you require help with dressing, washing, meals, etc., you can claim Attendance Allowance, and you can claim this even if there is no one looking after you.

Someone who stays at home to look after you and cannot go to work, may be able to claim Invalid Care Allowance.

If you have young children, and have no one to take them out each day while you rest, Social Services may be able to arrange a child minder for a few hours a day.

You can be assessed by someone from Social Services who will visit at home. When you are being assessed and questions are being asked, remember how you are *at your worst*, even if the visit takes place on one of your better days.

Be quite definite about how much disability the illness is causing. It is no good saying, 'Sometimes I can stand for long enough to wash up', if this is the exception rather than the rule. The problem with ME is in convincing people that your energy evaporates very quickly and is insufficient to provide for the most basic needs of living. You must describe yourself as you are at your worst, and not minimize or be apologetic about your disability. This advice also applies if you apply for Invalidity Benefit or Severe Disablement Allowance, or see a doctor for assessment for Mobility Allowance.

Local support services (mainly Social Services) can arrange occupational therapy, home helps, home visits by chiropodists, home aids, etc. The Social Service Transport Section organizes the Orange Badge parking scheme.

The Citizens Advice Bureau can advise on these and other services, and if necessary will visit you at home.

Registering Disabled

The Register of Disabled Persons was set up by the Manpower Services Commission to help disabled people to get employment.

You can apply for registration whether you are in employment or not. Registration is voluntary, but some facilities are only available to those who are registered.

Applicants will be asked to produce medical evidence to support their application, or have a medical assessment.

Registering as disabled with the MSC is not the same as registering with the Social Services. You can get further information from your local Job Centre. Various benefits from registering disabled with the MSC can include adaptations to help with your work, help with public transport, easier parking, and help with rehabilitation and training schemes.

Mobility

You can apply for an *Orange Badge* disabled car sticker if you cannot walk more than 50 yards. There may be occasional days when you *can* walk over 50 yards without detriment, but if the disability is the rule rather than the exception, apply for the badge. Application forms are supplied by the Social Service Transport Section, and will be posted to you in response to a phone call.

An Orange Badge can improve the quality of life enormously – visiting a bank, a hairdresser, the library, and friends whose houses are on yellow lines, all become possible. Otherwise the distance to such places from a car park may be just impossible on foot.

Mobility allowance

To be eligible you must be unable or virtually unable to walk, or have a condition in which walking seriously harms your health (e.g. heart disease or ME). It is not means tested, and is independent of other sources of income. Your local DHSS office will send the application form. You will normally be examined by a doctor who is not your GP. It takes about two months to come through, if your application is accepted. It is paid to help a disabled person run a car, or take taxis – i.e. to be mobile.

Summary of Benefits, April 1988

A useful booklet is *FB28 'Sick or Disabled?'* available from post offices and DHSS and Social Services offices. It has a list of other leaflets about specific services.

(1) Employed, and paid Class I National Insurance:
Statutory Sick Pay – up to 28 weeks, minimum 4 days
Invalidity Benefit – after 28 weeks

(2) Employed or self-employed, and paid National Insurance:
Sickness Benefit up to 28 weeks
Invalidity Benefit – after 28 weeks

(3) Unemployed, or not paid enough National Insurance contributions:
Income Support (used to be 'Supplementary Benefit')
Unemployment Benefit

(4) Unable to work for over 28 weeks, and ineligible for Invalidity Benefit, not paid enough NI contributions:
Income Support
Severe Disablement Allowance – if at least 80 per cent disabled
Mobility Allowance – unable to walk
Attendance Allowance – needing constant looking after
Invalid Care Allowance – the carer spending at least 35 hours a week looking after someone who gets Attendance Allowance.

Income Support is made up of:

- personal allowance;
- plus premium payment (for people with special expenses);
- plus possible housing costs payment.

The *Social Fund* helps with exceptional expenses.

Help with NHS charges is available for those on Income Support or low income: free NHS prescriptions, free NHS dental treatment, and help towards the cost of glasses.

Two other useful DHSS leaflets are *HB2 'Equipment and Services for Disabled People'* and *HB4 'Help with Mobility'*.

You do not have to go to a DHSS office to find out what help you are entitled to. Phone your local Social Security Office and ask to be sent the relevant leaflets, or write to P.O. Box 21, Stanmore, Middlesex, HA7 1AY.

The ME Association has produced two useful booklets, *A Guide to Benefits* and *A Guide to Services and Resources*. The latter describes the various services which exist in the community, outlines the main resources available to help ME sufferers and suggests ways of maximizing the chances of getting help.

To obtain these, and information about their cost, write, enclosing s.a.e., to the ME Association (address in Appendix A).

Wheelchairs

You do not need to be totally unable to walk to consider getting a wheelchair. A wheelchair, plus someone to push it, can open up horizons for you if you cannot walk very far. You can potter round a shopping centre, visit art galleries, stately homes, or go for an outing in your neighbourhood. Trips away, holidays, all sorts of outings may now be possible with a wheelchair. Apply to Social Services or the Red Cross for the loan of one.

Caution – do not wheel the chair yourself. ME affects the arms as well as the legs and the wheelchair is to conserve your energy! The helper who pushes you will need a few practice sessions away from a busy road or pavement. A common mistake for the learner-pusher is to allow the chair to tip forward when going off a pavement, risking the occupant falling out. To negotiate pavements, steps or bumps, the chair is tipped back so the weight is all on the main wheels. The other main rule in the wheelchair code is brakes on when parking the chair! Your pusher needs to be reasonably fit, as well as willing, for wheelchairs can be hard work especially on uneven ground.

Many ME patients whose walking is quite limited shy off from the idea of a wheelchair, because they do not want to become, or be seen as, an invalid. Being an invalid is partly a state of mind, and is a way other people perceive you. Better to see the wheelchair as a useful tool to help you get out of the house and join in the rest of the world at times. If you have a remission or get better, you won't need it.

Walking aids

The best aid, other than a wheelchair, is a folding stool-stick which can be used as a walking aid, then unfolds easily to a seat when needed. It is absolutely invaluable if you get tired aching legs when having to stand for any time. If you are half-way round a supermarket and feel dreadful and shaky, you can park yourself on the stool for a few minutes, also at the checkout, in queues at the bank, shops, bus stops and railway stations.

This gadget is *not* the same as a 'shooting stick', which has a sharp point to go into the earth, while watching birds fall out of the sky, and has a very small seat. These are quite unsuitable, as the sharp point will not stay put on a shop floor or pavement! The best stool-stick I have found is sturdy, with four non-slip rubberized 'feet', a strong canvas seat, and is made in different heights (32, 34, 37 and 39 inches).

They are obtainable from various retail outlets, including National Trust Centres, and some sports shops – those that supply things for hunting and shooting. (Address of a supplier in Appendix A.)

Travel

It is possible to go away on holiday with ME, but obviously not while acutely ill. For some, a change to sea or mountain air, the sun, and new horizons may be enjoyable and benefit the health. For others, especially those who get vertigo and visual problems from movement, the journey may be too comfortable, and the need to adapt to new surroundings and a new daily routine may be too much to cope with.

Air travel may seem quick and simple, but in practice it is the most stressful form of transport since the days of the bumpy stage-coach. If you decide to go for a holiday by air, it is wise to choose a time of year out of season, and to avoid those airports that are notorious for congestion or delays. It may actually be worth paying extra and travelling on a scheduled flight instead of a charter flight.

If you are unable to walk or to walk far – distances on foot at aircraft terminals may be 1/4 mile or more – ask the travel agent, or the airline direct, to arrange a wheelchair or buggy. This will then be organized again at the destination airport. This needs to be arranged *in advance*, and confirmed a day or two before travelling.

In theory this all sounds fine, but beware of Gatwick airport and its new terminal! Opened in 1988, modern, with arcades of dazzling shops and piped 'musack', the new terminal is a nightmare for the disabled, or indeed for anyone with a mountain of luggage and small children.

Wheelchairs and luggage trolleys are not allowed on the inter-terminal connecting monorail train – they have to be left behind about 30 yards before entering the train. If you are lucky, someone different will meet you with another wheelchair at the other end. If you have a lot of luggage, tough. It is quite hard to find another trolley when you leave the monorail train.

Having researched this airport and its new north terminal recently, when going on a holiday to Greece, I heartily advise against using it unless you can contact the airport authorities in advance and find out if the rules have changed or if they have now arranged means for a disabled person to arrive at the plane without having to change wheelchairs and walk!

The other disadvantage of air travel, apart from the stress and noise in airport terminals, is the level of chemicals in aeroplanes and terminals. If you are chemically sensitive, then you may feel quite unwell for a day or two after the flight. Some sufferers are adversely affected by the drop in pressure in the aircraft; this may particularly affect those with breathing problems.

Side effects of air travel, or any travel where

increased exposure to chemicals and stress happens, can be helped by taking extra vitamin C before and during the journey, 1 to 3 grams, and drinking plenty of water.

Travelling by train is probably better than air, or coach, or car on long motorways. British Rail issue Disabled Persons Railcards, which allow travel with 30 per cent reduced price tickets for both the holder and an escort. If you have Mobility Allowance or Severe Disablement Allowance, you can apply. If notified in advance, BR staff will help you on the train and meet you with a wheelchair or 'buggy' at the other end, which whisks you through the crowds in comfort to a taxi or a meeting car.

There is a useful leaflet, *British Rail and Disabled Travellers*, available from BR stations. If you do not drive, cannot afford to run a car, and do not have a carer or relative to drive you, then rail transport for long journeys is relatively painless, provided you ask BR for help at least a day in advance.

When travelling, and if using assistance, do not try even to walk a little way – the staff will not understand if you say you can walk a few yards but get tired. Just be totally disabled. The type of disability produced by ME is very difficult for most people to understand, especially as we don't have crutches or callipers.

A problem encountered by some in long car or coach journeys is that of petrol or diesel fume pollution entering the vehicle; this is worst of all on busy roads or in traffic jams. A car with a filter at the air intake may help, but these are rare. It may help to be aware of this problem, and close all windows and vents when in slow-moving traffic.

The decision on whether or not to travel, and how to travel, is a very individual matter. But the opportunity to travel and escape from four walls should not be dismissed out of hand. A journey will need much more planning and thought than it did when you were well, but is still possible. I know of at least two ME sufferers, both hardly able to walk, who have had enjoyable trips abroad with the help of a wheelchair, other people and schedules that still allowed plenty of rest.

House and Garden

There are lots of ways of making home life easier. Most energy saving ideas come from fellow sufferers, and in every copy of your national ME Society's newsletters you will find many helpful ideas. In the home, several obvious possibilities are:

- Have your bed on the same floor as the bathroom, if you are in a bed-resting phase.
- Do everything in the kitchen sitting down, if possible, by arranging a chair at a work surface for food preparation, and using a high stool at the sink for washing up, and raising the washing-up bowl to the same height.
- Collect everything that you need for preparing a meal in one container, e.g. in a washing-up bowl or basket, and take to the work area before sitting down.
- Iron sitting down, or do not iron at all; there is very little that really needs ironing, or cannot be ironed by someone else.
- If finance allows, consider investing in a machine that chops and mixes food, i.e. a food processor. Chopping vegetables can be exhausting, and the temptation would then be to live on toast and tinned food, which will not improve health.

- If you are spending a lot of time in bed, and are well enough to talk on the phone, get a phone extension (which you can switch off) by the bed There are telephone aids for disabled people; a shoulder rest to save you holding up the receiver is very helpful. Have a very comfortable armchair in the bedroom by a window, ask someone to fix a bird-table within view, and get some binoculars Make your bedroom cheerful, warm and homely to be in.
- In the bathroom, have a stool or chair to sit on while drying or undressing. If having a bath is too exhausting, a stool or chair under the shower is a solution. If there is no shower, try sitting on the stool in the bath, and have a bowl of warm wate on a chair next to the bath. Scoop the water ou with a large tin mug and slosh over you, or ask your helper to do this for you. You can wash al over and rinse while sitting down, and feel fresh and clean afterwards. In countries with limited water or no plumbing, this is the normal way to have a warm 'shower'!
- Make sure the bathroom is warm for the all-ove wash. This 'two chair and bowl' method is much less exhausting than a bath or standing by a basin A non-slip bath mat is essential for any method especially if you have problems with balance o co-ordination.
- In the garden, have a very comfortable seat at hand with leg rests, such as an adjustable sunbed, to li or rest on. Doing gentle gardening can be very therapeutic to the soul if one is well enough, and i gets one out of the house into fresh air and light but there must be somewhere to rest at frequen intervals. There is a gardening stool for disabled people available, which one sits in and can then

weed or use tools at ground level. A local garden supply centre should have details on such an aid. Even in a wheelchair, it is possible to work in raised beds and borders. Sowing and 'potting on' can be done in a greenhouse from a chair.

- The main enemy action in the garden is bending over or crouching, which places great strain on thigh and back muscles. Sitting on newspaper or other waterproof layers, beside a section of plant bed, is preferable.

Keeping Warm

Keeping warm is very important. In ME the circulation is usually bad, the body's thermostat doesn't work properly, and a lot of energy can be wasted in fighting the cold – energy which is needed for other vital functions. The problem is not confined to the winter, at least not in the UK, where temperatures can drop low enough to require heating, hot water bottles and electric blankets even in August.

Remember to keep the feet warm at all times, and that 30 per cent of the body heat is lost from the head. A woolly hat may be helpful, not only for outside, but in bed at night, or while inside in cold weather. Several thin layers of clothes are always better insulating than a few thick ones, and extra layers should always be at hand to put on wherever you are, especially if away from the house. A sudden feeling of chilliness can strike at any time, regardless of the weather, often due to a drop in blood sugar, or rapid exhaustion; the body temperature may bear no relation to whether you feel hot or cold! A sudden attack of iciness may mean you need to have something to eat, or have a sleep.

Just because others in the household may be comfortable in shirtsleeves, it doesn't mean that it is warm enough for you. But rather than turning the central heating up (70° F, 21° C, is the maximum advisable), you should wear more clothes and pay attention to head, feet and the neck. It is still important to have some ventilation in the home, even in cold weather.

In cold or chilly weather it is sensible to have a stock pot of soup or a stew on the go. This supplies instant hot food with minimal time to spend in a cold kitchen just before a meal. Certain foods have warming properties, such as ginger, cayenne pepper (caution – you only need a pinch), most curry spices, peppers, garlic, brown lentils. These foods will warm you whether they are taken hot or not, and are good to include in stews or soups.

Heated mini-blankets, or heat pads, are a good way to supply warmth to the back, chest or tummy as needed if you are cold with stiff or painful muscles. An electric blanket is marvellous for providing instant warmth when you get into bed, all the year round. Do make sure it is safe, though, and do not leave it switched on while in bed if it is an underblanket.

A warm bath or shower is good for warming, and also for improving circulation and lymph fluid flow, and for removing waste products that the body gets rid of through the skin via the sweat. Many people forget that the skin is an organ that eliminates toxins and body waste, so sweating a lot when you are ill is not a bad thing. The kidneys, skin, colon and lungs all get rid of waste, plus water, which needs to be replaced in ample amounts.

However a *hot* bath, one which is over 99° F or 37° C, is not recommended if you are ill, weak, or have any heart symptoms, because of the extra strain it puts on the circulation. Unless specifically advised as part of hydrotherapy treatment, a bath should not be above body temperature.

Part of the benefit of a bath or shower comes from a rub down all over when drying; this stimulates circulation of lymph, the fluid carrying the white cells. Drying yourself may be the most exhausting part of the washing process, you may need to ask for help with this if there is much muscle pain and fatigue. It's better to forget modesty and have some help, rather than forgo a regular bathe which does much good to morale and body.

Many important helpful hints have certainly been left out of this chapter. The best ideas come from other people whom you meet or telephone through local ME groups. As someone said, inventions are born of necessity! Only someone with the same problem as you, can really advise you how to solve it.

19

Children and ME

Children and adolescents can and do develop ME.

They can also suffer from the effects of ME in parent or sibling; they may feel left out, neglected o unloved if more attention is given to a sick brother o sister, or if an ill parent has not the energy for goo parenting. A child may suffer anguish at seeing parent devastated by ME; this may be demonstrate by bad behaviour or depression or sleep disturbance. am not going to write any more about child psychol ogy, but it is important to remember the silent suffer ing of a young child where another member of th family has severe ME, or any other chronic illness.

The onset of ME in a young person does not diffe from an adult, although it is usually acute, and follow an infection which is frequently present among schoo mates.

The clinical features and chief symptoms are n different from those experienced by an adult although some of the nervous system symptoms ma not be so obvious because a child is less likely t complain specifically of poor memory, poor con centration or depression.

Children tend to become ill rapidly if they develo an infection, and they will tend to have a highe temperature than adults and more severe symptom associated with the infection. They react more rapidl than adults, but also recover more quickly from mos acute infections. So it is noticeable when a youngste who has been laid low with fever, headache, mayb liarrhoea or vomiting and tummy pain, fails to make he expected recovery and be up and running around n a week or two.

Let us look at the problems of children with ME.

)iagnosis

'he agreed criteria for diagnosing ME include a ength of illness of six months or more. Clearly, arents are going to be concerned enough to want to now what is wrong before their child has been ill for ix months! Bearing in mind that physical activity nakes the condition worse, and that rest early on nay allow early recovery, it is obviously very important to get an assessment and provisional diagnosis vhen the child is not recovering as expected from an nfection – this may be a diagnosis of a 'post viral atigue syndrome' (PVFS), made on the basis of the istory and the absence of signs or tests for any other lisease.

Once this diagnosis has been reached, maybe as arly as six or eight weeks after the onset of illness, the hild can be allowed to rest as needed, the school is nformed, and pressure to go to school or do sports is emoved. The diagnosis may become ME if the illness ontinues for many months, with classical symptoms f muscle fatigue and brain disturbance.

Some GPs and school doctors are still reluctant to liagnose PVFS or ME in a child. They may either still onsider that ME is psychological, or believe that it is a ondition mainly experienced by the over-20s.

Although ME itself is less common under 20, very nany children suffer prolonged fatigue after an nfection, and some of these do continue unwell or ven deteriorate, and have the classic ME syndrome

for a year or more. It is tragic for a child and th
parents to have to battle with GPs and educatio
authorities for months, while the child may try t
attend school, to learn, and to live a normal life bu
keeps on relapsing and possibly deteriorates.

If your GP is ignorant about ME and other post vira
syndromes, or is simply unhelpful, you can do severa
things:

- (a) Contact the ME Association (address i Appendix A) and obtain information for th GP about the illness.
- (b) Change to another doctor
- (c) Find out if there is a specialist in your area wh understands ME, and ask for a referral, o make a private consultation.

Because there are often strange psychological symp
toms, and the fatigue leads to inability or reluctanc
to go to school or to do homework, some doctors an
education authorities find it easier to diagnose 'schoc
phobia' rather than suspect PVFS. They may also tr
to diagnose some 'family behaviour problem' t
explain the child's change in behaviour.

Factors which help in the diagnosis of PVFS/ME:

- A child who was enjoying school and sports ha *changed* since becoming ill – the psychologic problems are *new* and out of character.
- The association of what was obviously an acut infection with the onset of the illness.
- Worsening of the child's symptoms after exercis or after mental exertions – e.g. after sports or a te or exam.
- Fluctuating symptoms from week to week or da by day.

- Aches and pains quite unlike anything the child has had before.
- Symptoms not improved by going on holiday, or at weekends; in other words, normal family life and exercise out of school are just as bad as school activities. A child with school phobia would be expected to make a dramatic improvement during holidays!

Before the consultation with a GP or specialist, write down the history of the onset of the illness, and any of the above factors if they apply to your child.

Do not be fobbed off by a doctor if you think your child has PVFS. Insist that adequate tests are done to exclude other physical illnesses, and if there is no diagnosis, ask what else is making your child ill.

If the doctor does not know about ME, and finds no physical signs of illness, and blood tests are normal, the next stage may well be a referral to a child psychologist or psychiatrist. This assessment will be quite exhausting for the child, however many parents do agree to such an assessment; a properly trained and skilled psychologist should be able to conclude that the child with PVFS or ME has mental fatigue and signs of illness, rather than a purely psychological upset.

The results of such an assessment may actually strengthen your case.

Management of Children with PVFS and ME

Complete physical and mental rest must be encouraged at first. For the first few weeks or months, general nursing care as of any ill child is appropriate. The appetite may be poor, there may be nausea, constipation, diarrhoea, tummy pains, or seve headache. Do not use aspirin for pain; rather a sm dose of paracetamol, or homeopathic remedies if yo doctor uses them. Constipation seems to make sym toms worse, possibly due to toxins absorbed from t bowel, so encourage plenty of fluids, and as mu vegetable and fruit intake as possible – a liquidizer f making vegetable soups is invaluable.

Try and avoid sugar, 'junk food', coke and oth unnutritious things favoured by children. The di guidelines of Chapter 7 apply to children, and ad quate protein intake is especially important for weig to be maintained and growth to continue.

Problems arise when the child appears to ma some recovery and wants to do activities with friend or to go to school and behave normally. You cann force the child to stay in bed or in the house all t time, neither can you stand back and watch unco trolled behaviour which will inevitably lead to relapse.

The child's friends may be unsympathetic or ev cruel when they see their pal going to school for hal morning, looking quite normal, then having to home to rest for the remainder of the day. Keeping with the peer group is very important for children a teenagers, and the loss of friends and activities shar with them can be as damaging psychologically as t pain and other symptoms.

When the child is getting better enough to want go and do things, then a diary is a good idea, so t he or she can learn *for themselves* what the limits of t illness are at the time.

A frank discussion about the illness, what h caused it, how it affects the body and mind, and t probability of getting better, is a good idea at t stage. This will also dispel fears about other disea such as cancer or heart disease or leukaemia, which may be preying on a young mind. With TV programmes about illness abounding, youngsters may know a lot about disease and death at an early age.

A plan of rest and activity for the patient can be discussed among the whole family, so that the child is involved to some extent with managing the illness. Brothers and sisters and friends should be encouraged to include the patient in talking about what is going on in school and in their activities.

School, education

Hopefully, once you have a diagnosis, the school authorities will be understanding and co-operative about any restricted ability to attend school. There is a need for flexibility, and in some cases a compromise is needed so that part-time attendance is possible. Avoiding sports such as gymnastics, team games and athletics is mandatory until it is clear that improvement is virtually permanent.

Anyway, as with adults, children and students who have PVFS or ME will find that the less physical activity is undertaken, the more energy will be available for the brain. In other words, some mental functioning may be possible so long as there is no physical exercise.

In theory, a home tutor should be a useful solution for children who are well enough to do some learning but cannot cope with the stress and noise of a full classroom. In practice, home tutors are rather thin on the ground, and may not be easy to arrange.

Sometimes a parent may be able to supervise some work at home provided by the school, done at a pace the child can manage on an 'as and when' basis.

Thanks to the work of the ME Association, Education Directors and their Special Needs Advisers have all been sent information about ME. Information has also been sent to the Association of Clinical Psychologists and to the Advisory Centre for Education (ACE).

The Advisory Centre for Education is a national independent education advice service for parents of children at state schools. They can give advice about legal rights, the roles and powers of local education authorities; they can give advice and help about problems of families versus LEAs, and where necessary provide support for legal actions. Their address can be found in Appendix A.

In some areas, there may be enough families with ME to get together, so that affected children and adolescents can meet, or receive home tuition together.

It is enormously helpful for an affected youngster to have friends who have the same problems, even if the communication is by post. As with adult ME patients, the knowledge that there are others like you relieves the isolation.

At the moment, no one has come up with any magic cure for young ME sufferers. The basic principles of management are no different to those advised for adults. Nutritional supplements are beneficial, at a dosage about half of those suggested for adults. Multi-vitamin and mineral preparations for children are available, in chewable or liquid form, at most chemists and health food shops.

The disruption to schooling and social development which results from getting this illness as a child or adolescent is serious. At an age when things move on quickly, to have to drop out of life for a year or more can have long-lasting consequences. The pressures on youngsters to succeed – at sports, with classwork, O and A levels, university and now the new GCSE exams – are great, reflecting the intense competition for jobs that awaits school leavers and university graduates.

Perhaps it is not only the viruses which are causing ME in children. Perhaps the tragedy resulting from the disease in those worst affected is yet another by-product of a society which places so much emphasis on achievement and material possessions; a society in which the opportunities to attain these things are so restricted by high unemployment, and the demand for paper qualifications for virtually every job.

Case History

The following is a tragic case history, which will hopefully have a happy ending. Few children are as badly affected as this one, but young children *can* develop ME and remain ill for some years.

IAN'S STORY, TOLD BY HIS MOTHER

May 1986 – Ian fell ill the week after he returned from Wales with his primary school. He had funny lumps behind his ears and base of head, and felt sickly. His parents both developed the same bug.

In *August 1986* we were on holiday by the sea. Ian was very sick and had diarrhoea also, these stopped after 24 hours, but he was in bed for several days, as he began to feel achy and so tired.

When he got up again, we had a trip to the zoo, but this was a disaster. The walk up the drive from the car park to zoo was just too much, and Ian was exhausted and in tears with tiredness!! He *never ever* got back to his real self. Five weeks later he started his new school and settled well.

15 September – he was ill at school, burning up, headache, sore tummy and felt sick. After a few days I took him to the doctor who said his glands were still swollen, but if he felt like going to school next day it should be OK. At this time teachers and other pupils were all ill with the same thing.

Ian did not improve, he had bad headaches, sore throats, felt sick all the time, and sweated very heavily. He had very acidy smelling breath especially in the mornings. His appetite was very poor because of the nausea. He had tests for possible glandular fever, which were negative. Later he had more blood samples, and these showed there had been a huge virus infection.

13 November – we saw Dr B (paediatrician) for the first time at the hospital. *Ian had been ill now for six months*. He had a brain scan, which was normal, also more blood tests and for hepatitis.

Christmas 1986 – Ian began to lose his balance and started to drag his right leg. His legs seemed to be getting very weak, he still had nausea, and could not sleep.

1987 dawned – Ian was no better, and his legs were weaker.

9 February – we flew to Liverpool, where he'd been referred for a second opinion. We had a wheelchair and lift on and off the plane.

Ian was examined and had blood tests, X-rays, brain scan, EEG, etc. These were all clear, and when we saw the specialist, he said *Ian had post-viral fatigue syndrome*, and although this could be worse than the actual virus, he felt sure he would make a good recovery, and we could return home.

Back home Ian was prescribed Optimax (which we found out was for depression, and was not recommended for children), and also Motillium for nausea, but had so many side effects from these two drugs that we stopped them.

28 April 1987 – Ian still had all the symptoms, but was getting worse. The paediatrician said he couldn't help, and suggested we saw a psychiatrist, 'just to help keep his spirits up, with the illness going on so long'. Ian has never been *depressed*.

Our GP suggested some very gentle leg exercises to try to keep the muscles 'ticking over' for when he started to feel better. We only went to physiotherapy the first morning, as he found it so exhausting. We carried on with some of the exercises at home, but it made him feel more sick, tired and sore, and the bad breath came back, which had eased.

19 May – we took Ian to see Dr C (psychiatrist). He said that the virus which had affected Ian could be Coxsackie B, as this can cause disability like polio, but that you do get better from it. He also said, '*Only complete and utter rest* can cure, and it could take up to two *years*.'

In July we flew to Liverpool with Ian again for tests to be repeated. No tests were carried out, only examination by doctors. It took two doctors to support Ian if they tried to stand him up, as his legs would no longer hold him. One of the staff told him there was nothing wrong with him and he would be walking in two weeks. Ian said to us did he have to die to prove how ill he felt?

The Liverpool consultant felt it was a psychiatric problem, and that Ian would be better in a psychiatric place, removed from the environment in which he had become ill. We were told we would have the final say, so we did not accept the psychiatric treatment offered, and took him home.

Back at home Ian was admitted to our local hospital

to have the tests we had expected in Liverpool. But a 'few days' turned into a three week Hell.

The only test carried out was a lumbar puncture, which was normal. The first time we visited, we were told not to ask Ian how he was, and if he said he felt sick, or had a headache or anything, we were to ignore it and change the subject. They started giving him physio which made him feel really ill, and the pain in his back brought tears to his eyes. He was told not to be a baby!

Ian couldn't hold a spoon or fork as he couldn't grip any more, and could hardly lift his arms up. He was forced to feed himself; this would take him ages, and his food would go stone cold. His voice was getting weaker by now, and it was often too tiring for him to repeat something. He would tell us he couldn't put up with much more. Only we believed him, no-one else believed how ill he really felt.

Soon after this, we were given an article from a magazine called 'What is this scourge called ME?' There in black and white were all the symptoms our son had – mental confusion, headaches, sore throats, sickness, vivid dreams, heightened sensitivity to light and sound, etc. Here at last was the answer, we now felt we had found out what was wrong.

12 August 1987 – we went to see Dr Morgan-Hughes at the National Hospital, London, where after an hour's consultation and examination he said *Ian was a severe case of ME or post viral fatigue syndrome.* We were pleased to have a diagnosis. Dr M–H said it could be years before Ian was really better, that school was out for the foreseeable future, and that physio was wrong until he started to show an improvement; he would write this in his letters to the doctors at home.

End of September – Ian needed to have laxatives every

fourth night. He also started to cough with smoke, or car fumes, especially diesel from buses and lorries if they passed us on our walks in his wheelchair. Grass cuttings, perfumes, washing powders, etc. would make him sneeze, and set his body shaking as though his balance had gone. Also his voice became so weak, that it was just too exhausting for him to repeat anything. His fingers were now like a fist, and it was too painful to ease them out.

None of these things worried Ian, but we knew that the psychiatrist was just trying to get a response to his questions that would show that it was something in Ian's mind that was making him ill. We have always believed and still do that our son is physically ill, it is not in his mind, and we will go on and on fighting for him.

Mid October – Ian's right side would ache. He had huge ulcers on his lips. He still got confused if too many questions were asked at once. TV and flashing lights hurt his eyes. He had to wear darker tinted glasses. The doctors have never believed how sensitive to light and noise he has become.

One day the psychiatrist called, and amazed us by saying he *still* didn't believe Ian had ME . . .

We decided to take Ian privately again to see Dr Morgan-Hughes in London, as since August his voice had gone altogether, and he could no longer open his fingers.

21 March 1988 – we took Ian to the National Hospital in London again. Blood tests, brain scans, X-rays, EEGs, ECGs, etc. were carried out, and all were fine. All the doctors there said he had a 'physical and organic' illness, and always said he had ME.

We were asked to speak to a psychiatrist one day, who was doing research into people with ME. He never saw Ian. After telling him the history of Ian's illness, he told us 'children do not get ME'. We disagreed with him, but he insisted Ian did not have ME and he asked a top child specialist at Great Ormond Street Hospital (next door) to come. (This psychiatrist had not seen or examined our son.)

Next day the specialist from Great Ormond Street, a Dr L, came; he also did not examine Ian. After listening to our story of how Ian's illness had progressed over 18 months, he just said that he saw 12 children a year like him. We *thought* he meant children with ME but later had our doubts. He suggested a combination of medical and psychiatric treatment, in Great Ormond Street, the children's hospital, and Dr M–H could come over to keep an eye on us.

5 April – Ian was admitted to the metabolic ward in Great Ormond Street, to start speech therapy and physiotherapy. Another psychiatrist told us that the whole family needed to attend for 'family therapy' sessions. I explained this would be impossible because of the cost and distance from home. This doctor just couldn't accept this at all, and kept telling me that without these family sessions Ian would never get better. Also, that as a family we would not be able to cope with Ian getting better!

I said 'rubbish', if we, as a family could cope with our son becoming ill, I could assure them we could cope with him getting better.

Ian started treatment, the speech therapist would sit him in front of the computer for an hour. The bright green screen and the concentration would give him a bad headache. He then had to go for physio for over an hour, forced to stand for the whole time. He was shattered and ill when he came back from it.

We went to see the ward the psychiatrist wanted to put Ian in. The door had a combination lock on it, 'to keep the wrong people getting in, not the patients getting out' . . . Children sat in a classroom *glassy eyed* . . . and one girl was literally ripping her room apart. She was cowering in a corner screaming and swearing at the nurse.

It scared all of us, and we knew immediately it was not the place for a child so ill with ME.

Having seen the ward, we could only consider Ian being admitted if the following could be agreed in writing: 'No drugs without our consent, unlimited visiting by parents, use of ME diet, etc.'

Dr L was sorry we could not agree on the treatment, and said that we could take Ian back home, and arrange for him to have mild physio, speech therapy and counselling.

We flew back home. In the letter to our GP, it was said that we had discharged ourselves and 'kept denying Ian treatment'.

20 May 1988 – we took Ian to see Dr P, a well-respected homeopathic doctor. After a 2¼ hour private consultation with him *he* confirmed Ian still had ME and maybe some candida infection also. He gave us a diet to try, and also prescribed nystatin, and vitamins and minerals, and asked to see him again in one month's time. We came away feeling we were at last getting somewhere, but how mistaken we were . . .

Monday 23 May 1988 – our world came to an end . . . two social workers arrived on our doorstep, and *took Ian from us* under a 'place of safety order' – no warning, **nothing** . . . We weren't allowed to go in the ambulance with him, and did not even know when we would ever see him again. The order had been signed the day before (by a magistrate), and Ian was to be under the joint care of Dr C and Dr B (psychiatrist and paediatrician).

We were not allowed to see him for five days. Even now we still only have half an hour a day. When Ian was taken from us, even our parish priest was not allowed to see him. He was angry, and said he didn't think priests or vicars were *ever* stopped from seeing anyone in hospital! Thank God, later our vicar was allowed in to see Ian, he was our *only* link till we saw him.

He was alone in a ward, could not move at all, could not speak, and had no way of getting help if he needed it. He had been told he had been taken from us because he was dying, and he sat waiting to see us with that bottled up inside him.

One day a doctor told him: 'There is nothing wrong with you, if you don't talk next week, you will be better off in our Mental Home, and never go home again.' Ian was so scared, he wet himself as he sat in his wheelchair (which he had never done while ill). And there were other threats to make him walk and talk, e.g. 'if you don't talk we will stop your parents' visits'.

They still maintained that he did not have ME and they were just trying to scare him into talking and walking. One night we found him very upset – he had wet himself, as no one had asked him if he needed the toilet. At home he had a bell to use to call us; even in the other wards, where patients could walk and talk, they still had a 'call' button.

Friday is the day he always dreads, as he goes to a remedial pool, and one day they let him go, certain he would put his arms out to save himself; he couldn't, so he went right under the water. The terror that child felt must have been indescribable. We have tried in vain to get the swimming stopped.

We are not allowed near him at meal times, the staff cannot discuss anything about Ian with us. He looks shattered each night on days he has had physio. His mouth is full of nasty ulcers again, his constant headaches are back, but no one ever asks him how he feels, so they never know. The nausea is much worse, and his eyes hurt because they removed his dark glasses. The noise of the other children is too much at times due to his heightened sensitivity to noise.

When he was in the National Hospital, London they fitted his hands with splints, to open the fingers slowly, and you could straighten them and bend them for him easily. Now he hardly has his splints on, so his fingers are bending up again.

Dr C now says Ian has never had ME. It's just school phobia, and an over-protective mother.

We were told in London by a psychiatrist, who never even saw Ian, that children *do not get ME*. He was supposed to be an expert in the illness too . . .

Our latest hope in our battle to have our son returned to us, is the visit we have had of a paediatrician from Wales. He examined Ian, had a long talk with us,and said that *Ian has had ME and still has ME* . . .

August 1988 – now we have to wait and see if the doctors here will at long last accept the diagnosis, or do we still have to go and fight it out in court to get our son back home. We have the constant fear at the back of our minds that if we lose at the end of it all, Ian will be put in a locked psychiatric ward, which we know is the wrong place for someone so very ill with ME.

[On 20 October 1988, after four months in hospital removed from the care of his parents, Ian was at last released back to his family. His condition was unchanged from May, if anything he was worse. A neurologist, Professor Field, had been allowed to examine Ian in September. His conclusion was that the child was a severe case of ME and that neither psychiatry nor hospital had any place in his treatment.

Now Ian is receiving treatment again from a homeopathic doctor, and his family wish to forget the nightmare and concentrate on helping him get better.]

20

Caring and Relationships

The illness of any member of a family inevitably adds to the strain of relationships in the group. If someone has an acute illness, or an injury, or an operation, there is an expectation that he or she will get better after a predicted period of convalescence, and will return to more or less normal life. So the period of upheaval is seen as temporary, it has some sort of boundary; the illness or operation is usually definable and recognized, and the whole period of illness and recovery can often be coped with.

But if having ME is, for the sufferer, a sentence of indeterminate length with no remission for good behaviour, it may be an equally long sentence for the person closest to the patient.

A lot of the difficulties that result from an ME patient trying to adjust to living at home and in the community rather than in hospital or nursing home, also apply to other chronic disabling conditions. The strain of caring for and loving someone with heart disease, MS, a stroke, kidney disease, epilepsy and cerebral palsy (and there are many others) is no different from that of caring for a badly affected ME sufferer.

However, what makes the ME syndrome different is the *variability* and *unpredictability* of both the physical state and the mood. As a carer, one day you may rejoice to see the patient happily pottering gently in the garden, the next day may find you helping with dressing and washing. One day there are hours of desperate sobbing and anguish, the next there is a calm person who cannot realize what a dreadful day they gave you yesterday.

The unpredictability of ME makes planning for the future difficult. By the time the diagnosis is made, the sufferer has probably been unwell for six months or more. Can one confidently go ahead with plans that affect the household such as moving house, holidays, renovations, job changes, another six months hence?

The fear of the future is always worse than the reality of the day. There is probably a better chance of peace of mind if no long-term plans are made which cannot be unmade; living from day to day and letting the future take care of itself is to some extent a good philosophy for ME families.

In reading any piece of writing about relationships, the assumption may be that a man-woman relationship is referred to. I am taking relationships to include those between friends, neighbours and other relatives, as well as immediate family. By 'carer', I mean the person or persons most closely involved with providing practical and emotional support for the ME patient.

In any close relationship, there is a tendency for the emotional mood of one to have an effect on the other.

If one person is sullen, withdrawn or depressed, the other thinks, 'What have I done to cause an upset?' It is so natural to take the emotional moods of a loved one as a reflection of how they feel about us, and so very difficult to be a detached, though caring, observer.

So if you are a carer, try and remember that your patient's rapid emotional changes are due to the illness, and not because of changed feelings to you or to a diminished need of you.

Because the life of the carer may be disrupted a

well as that of the sufferer, this can lead to resentment on the part of the carer, and guilt for the sufferer. But both sides try desperately not to let these quite natural feelings show. Guilt at being 'such a burden to you' is terribly common, and of course it just adds to all the mental suffering already experienced. The assurance of being loved and valued as a member of the household, in spite of being an apparently useless wreck, can reduce the guilt quite a lot.

The resentment felt by someone at having their life disrupted by this interminable illness in the patient is a common emotion, and should not be underestimated. And the person who is resentful then feels guilty about it, cannot express it for fear of upsetting the patient, so ends up irritable and moody. It is in this situation that an open loving relationship between carer and patient can deteriorate. You as a carer may experience feelings of anger, resentment, frustration, or grief because a loved one is ill and you don't know when he or she is going to get better; because both your lives are turned upside down; and because you, the carer, may have to sacrifice job, time, hobbies and holidays in order to be able to care effectively.

These feelings are perfectly normal, you are not Florence Nightingale or one of the saints! What is wrong is to bottle everything up and do damage to both yourself, the patient and other members of the household.

The ME Association in the UK provides valuable support for sufferers through local groups, and a 'listening ear' telephone service. But carers need support as well, and it may be helpful to talk to other carers, to people in the ME Association, or to anyone offering a sympathetic ear, if you feel you can't cope with ME and the patient.

Sadly, a number of relationships do break down

completely under the stresses created by ME, leading to separation, divorce, broken engagements, loss of lover or close friend, or children leaving home. I do not have the necessary skills to advise how to prevent these separations; they happen to many people without ME, but are harder to bear if a chronic illness is the main reason for the split.

Sometimes a relationship has been going wrong anyway, before ME appeared, and in such cases a severance may remove a major stress, and allow the patient a better chance to get better. However, sometimes the human resources of loving and understanding develop in two people as a result of one of them getting ME, and a lukewarm relationship may then grow into a much deeper and warmer one.

Possibly one of the most important aspects of some relationships to suffer is the sexual one. I do not think that a lessening of sexual desire is something confined to ME, but may be a symptom present with many chronic illnesses. After all, becoming ill is a sign that the whole body–mind complex is not functioning properly.

A sick animal or child rests, following the bodily need to conserve energy for healing. A sick adult human also stops expending energy on unnecessary activities. Sometimes there is not enough energy for digestion or for conversations, so the body is certainly not going to give much priority to the act of lovemaking! In women who are ill, loss of interest in sex is also a protective mechanism (unconscious) against becoming pregnant at a time when the body would be unable to cope with it.

It is easy to foresee that a previously stable marriage or loving relationship will become quite strained if one partner says, 'I'm too tired for it', for months or years.

The loss of sexual desire is a very common symptom

with ME, but is not something that people talk about readily to the family doctor. There are of course other ways of expressing affection as well as the sexual act itself. Some couples may succeed through compromise, such as finding occasions when the fatigue is not so great; using different techniques or positions; or perhaps by accepting that this one part of the relationship may have to be put aside for some time. Mutual understanding of why the problem arises, and accepting it as just another activity to forgo for a while – just as one has to accept that long walks, late nights, socializing, etc., are activities to be postponed until the patient feels better – is the main way to cope with this problem.

It is enormously helpful for the ME patient if the carer can demonstrate that he or she believes the patient has a genuine illness, and at the same time demonstrate the belief in possible recovery. It can be a bit difficult to draw the line between being supportive and helping in every aspect of living when needed, and in encouraging the patient to be an invalid.

There are times when the patient needs to be allowed to stretch the wings and try and do a bit more, and times when the carer needs to be firm and say, 'That's enough, you must rest.' Balancing the functions of a protective nurse with those of an occupational therapist can be tricky even when looking after a patient with an illness which is predictable. With ME, playing it just right, when your patient is so unpredictably up and then down, is nearly impossible.

Here is some advice to the ME carer, given by someone with experience of this challenging job!

- You must have patience, compassion, resilience and belief in ME as a mentally and physically crippling disease in varying degrees.

- You have to learn not to mind when people tell you you are being exploited by waiting hand and foot on someone who usually looks perfectly fit, e.g. in a wheelchair one week, and next week walking.
- You need to be aware of the varying limitations of the ME patient and be ready to step in, e.g. rescue patient from long and exhausting telephone conversations.
- You must be prepared to help in all aspects of daily living as required.
- If the ME patient, in desperation, behaves out of character, you must not take it to heart, and must learn not to be thrown by wide mood swings.
- Try to maintain the fine line between having a life of your own and yet still realizing the extent you are needed for moral as well as physical support.
- **In short – be a perfectly perfect person!!**

Carers often feel isolated, and need help and support. Most people in the UK do not know exactly how the Health and Social Services work; if you, or the person you look after, need outside help, you may not know how to go about asking.

There are three sources of help to try first:

(1) *Your family doctor*
Do not neglect to tell your GP about your own health problems – a sick carer is entitled to medical help just as much as the patient. Ask about any help which may be needed with lifting, dressing, bathing.

A district nurse may be asked to call and give advice.

(2) *The hospital*
If the ME sufferer is in hospital or attending outpatients, ask the specialist to explain any disabilities.

Many ME patients may prefer to avoid hospitals, as not all doctors and nursing staff understand what the llness is, and may want to institute physiotherapy.

Hospitals on the whole are *not* good environments as regards getting plenty of sleep and avoiding chemicals!

3) *Social Services*

The phone book gives the address and number of your local Social Services. You can ask

a) for a social worker to visit the home to find out the patient's needs;
b) for information about what is needed;
c) what home help is available.

There are carers' groups in many areas. The ME Association may know of some, or else your local Social Services or Citizens' Advice Centre, or local voluntary services may know of one.

Useful addresses for carers are given in Appendix A.

Case History

This last case history is of someone I have met.

The short story cannot adequately describe the courage and patience of the sufferer, nor the dedicated love and care of her family.

CLARE'S STORY

In December 1986, Clare was a second year university student, doing Psychology and English Literature. She lived in a Hall of Residence, was generally fit, enjoyed dancing and other active pursuits. On the morning of 6 December she woke with what seemed to be flu. She returned home to her parents' house, spent eight days in bed and felt exhausted. However, she seemed to recover, did her end of term exams and felt reasonably well over Christmas.

The flu returned on 2 January 1987 and, because she felt so exhausted, she went to the doctor on 6 January. The GP took a blood test which showed a high antibody titre to Coxsackie B virus. Clare then returned to hall, feeling decidedly more tired and much slower in her actions, some nights having to go to bed after tea. There was another visit to the doctor and another blood test – this time it showed negative antibody. In the meantime Clare's mother had read about ME and asked if this was a possibility. The GP totally rejected this, told Clare she had a post-viral condition, that she should continue with her studies but not take any strenuous exercise ('Aerobics maybe, but squash no!').

During the period from February to the end of the second term, Clare's condition worsened with a few brief spells of remission. She had greatly slowed down, couldn't imagine walking very far and was generally behind with her studies. During the Easter holidays she decided that she could no longer con tinue as a student and notified the university authori ties on 23 April 1987.

Around this time her GP referred her to a consultan at Ruchill Hospital who gave her a diagnosis of Pos Viral Fatigue Syndrome or ME and estimated that i might take anything up to three years to get better Gradually Clare ceased to be able to get up for meals She began to experience what she called 'a wobbl head' – a frightening feeling where the brain seems t be losing contact with the eyes. As well as the intens fatigue other symptoms appeared in the followin months – cold, almost wet feet, a sensitivity to light with after images, sensitivity to sound combined with a ringing in the ears culminating in a severe and constant headache in September.

Any kind of stimulation seemed to produce pain for her. She was no longer able to tolerate visits from friends and only limited contact with her family. Having a bath or hair washing was beyond her. She suffered intense malaise and often felt that she was dying. From this time on, her mobility disappeared and she had to be pulled to the bathroom on an office chair. Some days she was unable to sit up for meals and had to be fed.

During this period Clare's parents in increasing desperation sought help from various sources. A herbalist recommended an anti-candida diet which after five days made her feel very sick and caused vomiting. It also made her lose half a stone which, combined with the loss of muscle bulk, left her weight at seven stone. She discontinued the diet as she felt unable to cope with the nausea and further loss of weight.

A three-day stay in a homeopathic hospital in July was equally unsuccessful. She returned home with a promise to the doctor-in-charge to continue on a wheat-free diet for some six weeks (which she did) and to try and sit on a chair for ten minutes per day which she was unable to do. A physiotherapist was sent from the local hospital but even sitting out on a chair for more than a few seconds caused her to break out in severe sweating so this was discontinued.

Autumn 1987 and the symptoms were at their worst. She lay all day, every day, in a room with the curtains drawn and with wax plugs in her ears. An eczema type rash developed on her face and was only kept at bay by daily applications of cortisone cream.

The encephalitic symptoms were predominant – constant severe head pain, a sense of unreality, nightmares. Another homeopathic doctor, whose speciality was 'psionic medicine', was contacted. In all telephone calls and letters he promised 'a significant return to health in the very near future'. After three months and no sign of recovery Clare's disillusionment was intense. Reflexology was equally futile.

In January 1988 Clare was able to have the curtains opened – an hour a day initially, then throughout all the short winter days. She also decided to dispense with all diets, with keeping her food balanced and additive free. There was no proof that they helped and her life was restricted enough (the exception to this was not eating chocolate, which she found had a bad effect). During March/April her headaches were as bad as ever although sensitivity to noise had reduced.

In April 1988 she heard that injections of Parentrovite were being tried with some success by an immunologist in Belfast. With the agreement of her GP Clare has now had six fortnightly injections which do seem to have helped her condition somewhat.

She can now, in August 1988, watch television for short periods, listen to the radio, have a bath and hair wash once a week. She no longer needs her ear-plugs and can cope with much more family input. The headaches and the ringing in the ears are still there but are more intermittent and not so severe. This improvement was not dramatic but rather imperceptible on a day-to-day basis.

For the last five weeks she has been taking amitriptyline, one of the tricyclics, to combat panic attacks and because a recent *Horizon* television programme suggested that it might be useful in some ME cases. Initially there were some side effects but these were outweighed by an overall improvement in her condition

However after a year and a half in bed Clare is still unable to walk more than five steps, and her full recovery is a long way off.

21
Conclusion

In this book I have given an overview of the illness known variously as myalgic encephalomyelitis, chronic fatigue syndrome, once as epidemic neuro-myesthenia, and probably other names I may not have heard of. It is still quite a mystery disease to most doctors; probably those most knowledgeable about ME are the sufferers themselves. There is more to learn about it every day, and it is important that ME people communicate with each other about things that help, and continue to support research and the education of non-believers. It is hard to believe this in 1988, but people afflicted by multiple sclerosis had to battle for years to have their illness accepted as being genuine. Many of them were regarded as malingerers or neurotic twenty or so years ago.

Perhaps one day there will be a 'treatment' for ME, some medicine to take, some magic bullet to make it all better. Predictably, the main focus of current medical research into treatment is looking at ways of destroying the virus, or of sorting out the badly functioning immune system. This is fine, so long as the basic principles of helping the self-healing process are also applied – rest, good food, fresh air and light, freedom from stress and spiritual well-being.

In the USA, several therapies being investigated include:

(1) *Immunoglobulin (Gammaglobulin)*, given by intra-venous injection. This seems logical in those

cases where there is a lack of this antibody, and some trials in Australia suggest about 66 per cent show improvement. The usefulness of gamma-globulin is not yet proven in the UK.

(2) *Transfer Factor*. This, one of the immune system products, occurs naturally, and is expected to improve numbers and function of most white cells.

(3) *Ampligen*. This 'is a synthetic RNA, a pretend virus, which mimics the RNA in the immune system', and is said to be anti-virus and immune boosting.

(4) *Intravenous Vitamin C*. This is used by a few doctors; 50 grams of vitamin C are given at one treatment. In theory it gives a great surge to the immune system; in practice it is very expensive and not readily available. There is no evidence yet from trials of how useful it is.

(5) Some herbs, *Echinacea* and *Lomatium*, which are immune stimulants, are being investigated in the USA.

Further research needs to be organized, to look at various possible factors in the cause and incidence of ME. These would include geographical location, season, family history, occupation; details on housing, diet, exposure to chemicals; details of past drugs treatments, especially antibiotics; immunizations, amalgam fillings; and perhaps personality. All these things come under the heading epidemiology, which means literally 'the study of epidemics'. Some research into a possible hereditary predisposition to ME would also be very interesting.

In this book you will have noticed there is a word that is hardly used – that is the word CURE. Perhaps you are disappointed, having hoped to find guidance to lead you to the magic remedy that will make you fit, and full of energy to live the life you used to enjoy. Of course there *are* quite a number of ME people who get so much better that they consider themselves cured.

However, the possibility of relapse is always there, and it is really foolish for someone who seems to have recovered to push their body to the limits, or to go without sleep, or eat badly. The viruses that trigger off ME are still around, either gone back to sleep (become latent) in your body, or floating around in the community.

It is useful for anyone who has a chronic illness to consider the two terms 'health' and 'fitness', because we tend to think they are the same thing!

What is meant by being 'fit'? This is a state that is desired by athletes, by people who want to be able to do hard exertion without ill effects, and requires perfectly working heart, lungs and muscles. Fitness describes a purely physical condition, and ignores the state of the mind and the soul.

Health has a much more subtle meaning. I understand it to mean being integrated, balanced in oneself, at peace with the world and content. A state of 'perfect health' – if it exists! – would mean perfect function of body, and mind, and a pure spirit. In ME the body does not function properly, certainly, but I do believe that there is more to health and life than a super-fit or even half-fit body.

I know two quite different people:

Mr Super Fit takes great care of his body, he runs or plays squash every day, goes ski-ing and rock climbing (both to top levels of endurance) at weekends and holidays. In his forties, he has the body of someone much younger. However, he is unhappy, tense, gets lots of headaches and vague symptoms, is antisocial, irritable and sometimes depressed.

Mr Laid Back is also in his forties, he is a bit overweight, enjoys his food and some wine. He loves his job of teaching young children, loves entertaining friends, is generous and usually cheerful. Apart from walking and standing all day at school, and pottering in the garden, he takes no exercise whatsoever, and does not feel the need for it. He has not had a cold or day off work for years and does not have any bodily symptoms.

Which of these men is the healthier? And which of them would cope better with getting ME?

As stated earlier on, health means 'wholeness'. The ME stricken body may not be whole, sometimes it seems as though every part of it is broken down. But I am continually amazed at the wholeness of the spirit and personality of people I come across who are physically disabled in some way.

I can still vividly recall a patient I knew in a cancer and chemotherapy unit. She was only 38, her family were still young; she had an incurable cancer, was wasted and in a lot of pain. She had plenty to be resentful about, and to be scared of. Yet, following some sessions of healing with her parish priest, and knowing that many people were praying for her, she announced one day that she was healed. Her body did not miraculously rid itself of the cancer overnight; to a casual observer she still seemed desperately ill. What changed was that she accepted her condition, stopped being afraid, and felt completely at peace with her family, friends and her Maker. In her last few weeks of life she gave out so much love to those around her that those of us caring for her felt enriched by her company. In one sense this lady was healed and healthy.

So I think that one of the keys to getting on with ME is *acceptance* of how you are. This is not the same as wallowing in self-pity and saying, 'I'll never be any better.'

No, it means saying, 'ME has come into my life, it is a fact of life. I shall do what I can to improve the way I feel. I shall change my lifestyle, feed my body well, nourish my immune system, and give myself lots of tender loving care. I shall stop yearning for what I cannot have for the present, and count what blessings I do have. If I listen to my body and look after myself I shall probably get quite a lot better in time. If I do not get back to how I used to be, I will nevertheless continue to be alive and able to appreciate many good things in life, by living from day to day and looking for joy in very little things.'

Those who cope best with ME seem to be the people who try to go along with it, who adapt to living with ME, rather than fighting it. Ironically, there are other illnesses that one fights to get the better of – there is the saying 'fighting for life' in a severe infection or after an accident perhaps. But with ME one needs to be a bit less aggressive about the illness. There is a need for fortitude and resolution, certainly, and some discipline about *not* doing things. Because nobody who has ME ever knows exactly when they are going to get better, it is very important to be able to get on with some sort of life, even if it is only 10 per cent of the amount of living there was before.

So if it takes one week to complete a task, such as writing a letter, that used to take 20 minutes, never mind. The work done will have no less value!

Living with an illness such as ME is possible at all levels of affliction. Remember it does not kill, and that the majority do get better, and many improve in time. Whether or not you have any religious faith, you can appreciate that this prayer of St Francis of Assisi is one for ME people to learn and use:

> God, grant me the serenity
> to accept the things I cannot change,
> courage to change the things I can,
> and the wisdom to know the difference.

Appendix A

The ME Association

The ME Association was formed in 1976 by a small group of ME sufferers. It has now grown into a large and professionally organized charity with local branches existing all over the UK. Membership passed 12,500 in August 1988.

The association has three objectives – to find and offer support to sufferers, to spread information on the illness, and to promote medical research. A newsletter, issued every quarter, gives up-to-date information including current research, medical information, news nationally and from the local groups, and members' articles and letters.

The association has helped fund several research projects in different medical specialities. It gives support of great value to ME sufferers through its central office and the activities of local groups. A confidential telephone help line, 'Listening Ear', is manned by volunteer counsellors who are themselves sufferers.

The association has actively campaigned for and achieved government recognition of ME. In order to promote greater understanding in primary health care, it has undertaken the circulation of diagnostic information to all GPs. Information packs have been sent to a wide range of professional and voluntary agencies with which sufferers may come into contact. These include government departments, Directors of

Education and Social Services, disability groups, trade unions, professional associations, and information services.

It provides individual support for those seeking benefits and services. It has brought attention to those with special needs such as children with ME.

The association acts as a lifeline for those who are isolated, despairing, confused and devastated by ME. For many sufferers, the first positive development comes when they find they are not alone, that they do have a real illness (even if this is not recognized by their doctor), that others have similar experience and are there to offer friendship, encouragement and hope.

The address to write to – enclosing an s.a.e. please – is:

The ME Association, P.O. Box 8, Stanford-le-Hope, Essex, SS17 8EX.

The ME Action Campaign

The ME Action Campaign was formed in the summer of 1987. The founders of the campaign felt that a more dynamic and forceful approach was required to achieve recognition of ME by the government and medical profession.

In practice, this meant highlighting the plight of ME sufferers through the news media, and putting pressure on the government through Parliament to bring about recognition of the disease. This was achieved with spectacular success, mainly as a result of the involvement of Clare Francis, president of the campaign.

Due to the efforts of the campaign, Jimmy Hood,

MP for Clydesdale, presented the ME Sufferers Bill to Parliament on 23 February 1988. The Bill asked for an annual report to Parliament on progress made in investigating ME, and gained a great deal of publicity for the disease.

The Action Campaign's philosophy is that sufferers should not rely exclusively on the medical profession to solve their problem, but should be responsible for their own health, and take whatever steps are necessary to improve their situation. The campaign feels that alternative or complementary medicine has as much to offer the person with ME as conventional medicine, and acts as a source of information on the wide range of therapies and treatments that have helped people with the disease, whether or not they have been 'scientifically proven'.

The campaign is establishing a network of 'action groups' nationwide. These groups will provide support for people with ME, will inform local people through the press, radio and TV, and will raise funds.

The Action Campaign is also putting together a research programme, geared towards treatments that help patients, part of which will be carried out with the active involvement of the Institute of Complementary Medicine.

The new 80-page ME journal, called *Inter Action*, is being launched by the Action Campaign, and will contain a broad range of news, views and opinion, and covering the whole spectrum of medical expertise, conventional and alternative.

For an up-to-date factsheet on ME, which includes details of other information available from the campaign, simply send an s.a.e. marked 'Factsheet' to:

The ME Action Campaign, P.O. Box 1126, London, W3 0RY.

Other Useful Addresses

Outside the United Kingdom

ANZMES (NZ) Inc.,
P.O. Box 35–429,
Browns Bay,
Auckland 10,
New Zealand.

ANZMES Geraldton (Australia),
93 Ainsworth Street,
Geraldton,
Western Australia 6350.

ANZMES Victoria,
P.O. Box 7,
Moonee Ponds,
Victoria 3039,
Australia.

ANZMES Perth,
P.O. Box 293,
West Perth,
Western Australia 6005.

ANZMES N.S.W.,
P.O. Box 645,
Mona Vale,
New South Wales 2103,
Australia.

New Guinea ME Society,
P.O. Box 44,
Ukarumpa,
Via Lac,

Papua,
New Guinea.

Dutch ME Foundation,
P.O.B. 23670,
1100 E.D. Amsterdam S.O.,
Netherlands.

Norges ME Forening,
Gullerasveneien 14B, 0386,
Oslo 3,
Norway.

CFIDS,
Chronic Fatigue and Immune Dysfunction Society
1401 East Seventh Street,
Charlotte,
NC 28204,
USA.

CFSS,
Chronic Fatigue Syndrome Society
P.O. Box 230108,
Portland,
Oregon 97223,
USA.

UK societies; suppliers of specialized items

ARMS,
Action for Research into Multiple Sclerosis,
4a Chapel Hill,
Stanstead,
Essex, CM24 8AG. Tel: 0279 815553

Action Against Allergy,
43 The Downs,
London, SW20 8HG. Tel: 01 947 5082

Biolab,
The Stone House,
9 Weymouth Street,
London, W1N 3FF. Tel: 01 636 5959/5905
(for assessment of nutritional status, doctor's referral needed)

Society for Environmental Therapy,
3 Atherton Road,
Ipswich,
Suffolk, IP4 2LD.

British Society of Allergy and Environmental Medicine,
34 Brighton Road,
Banstead,
Surrey,
SM17 1BS. Tel: 07373 61177

British Dental Society for Clinical Nutrition,
Glenrose,
Bernards Close,
Great Missenden,
Bucks. Tel: 02406 4601/5997
(for information about testing for mercury sensitivity, etc.)

ACE Advisory Centre for Education,
18 Victoria Park Square,
London, E2 9PB. Tel: 01 980 4596

Disabled Living Foundation,
380–384 Harrow Road,
London, W9. Tel: 01 299 6111

MIND,
22 Harley Street,
London, W1. Tel: 01 637 0741.
(gives legal advice on rights of mentally ill patients)

Samaritans,
17 Uxbridge Road,
Slough, SL1 1SN. Tel: 0753 32713

National Federation of Spiritual Healers,
Old Manor Farm Studio,
Church Street,
Sunbury-on-Thames,
Middlesex, TW16 6RG. Tel: 0932 83164/5

National Institute of Medical Herbalists,
148 Forest Road,
Tunbridge Wells,
Kent, TN2 5EY. Tel: 0892 30400

British Homeopathic Association,
27a Devonshire Street,
London, W1N 1RJ.
(doctors trained in homeopathy)

Society of Homeopaths,
47 Canada Grove,
Bognor Regis,
West Sussex, PO21 1DW.

Transcendental Meditation,
Peel House,
Peel Road,
West Pimbo,
Skelmersdale,
Lancs, WN8 9PT. (Tel: (Freephone) 0800 269 303

Colonics International Association,
26 Sea Road,
Bascombe,
Bournemouth,
Dorset BH5 1DF

Henry Doubleday Research Organization,
Convent Lane,
Braintree,
Essex.
(advises on all aspects of organic gardening, and has a list of suppliers of organic produce)

The Soil Association,
86 Colston Street,
Bristol,
Avon.

Philips of Axminster,
Philips House,
West Street,
Axminster,
Devon EX13 5NX. Tel: 0297 32701
(supplier of walking stick stools)

Wholistic Research Company,
Bright Haven, Robins Lane,
Lolworth,
Cambridge, CB3 9HH.
(suppliers for VDU protective screens)

Bach Flower Remedies Ltd,
Dr E Bach Centre,
Mount Vernon,
Sotwell,
Wallingford,
Oxon, OX10 0PZ.

Becpharm Ltd,
London, E18 2LY.
(supplier of nystatin powder BP)

Renahall Ltd,
61 Lime Tree Avenue,
Rugby, CV22 7QT. Tel: 0788 811454
(supplier of vitamin C powder)

Lamberts Dietary Products Ltd,
1 Lamberts Road,
Tunbridge Wells,
Kent, TN2 3EQ. Tel: 0892 46488
(Lamberts products are obtainable on prescription through Boots chemists)

Nature's Best Health Products Ltd,
P.O. Box 1,
Tunbridge Wells,
Kent, TN2 3EQ.
(supplements as Lamberts; this address is for direct order by patient, not on prescription)

Probiotics

(a) **Green Farm Nutrition Centre,**
Burwash Common,
Etchingham,
East Sussex, TN19 7LX. Tel: 0435 882482
(to order Probion)

(b) **York Medical Supplies,**
4 Museum Street,
York, YO1 2ES. Tel: 0904 52378
(to order Vitaldophilus)

(c) **G+G Supplies,**
51 Railway Approach,
East Grinstead,
Sussex. Tel: 0342 230161
(to order Superdophilus)

Bio-Oil Research Ltd,
The Hawthorns,
64 Welsh Row,
Nantwich,
Cheshire, CW5 5EU.
(to order Naudicelle, a brand of evening primrose oil)

Britannia Health Products Ltd,
Forum House,
41–75 Brighton Road,
Redhill,
Surrey, RH1 6YS.
(to order Efamol, a brand of evening primrose oil; both of the above may supply a bulk order of evening primrose oil at a discount)

Note: There are also many good dietary supplements available in chemists and health food shops; the best are gluten, sugar, milk and additive free – look at labels.

Useful advice for people who care for the chronically sick or disabled

National Carers Association,
9 Chilworth Mews,
London, W2 3RG. Tel: 01 724 7776

Association of Crossroads Care,
Attendant Schemes Ltd,
94 Coton Road,
Rugby,
Warwickshire, CV21 4LN. Tel: 0788 73653
(both these are voluntary organizations offering support services for carers and their dependants)

Useful leaflet for carers

'Taking a Break – a guide for people caring at home' (produced by King's Fund). Free to carers, 60p to others, from

Taking a Break,
Newcastle upon Tyne X, NE85 2AQ.
(this leaflet gives information about ways in which those who care at home full-time for a chronically sick or disabled person can themselves obtain a rest, or break)

Appendix B

Other Conditions to be Excluded – Differential Diagnosis

Myesthenia Gravis
Polymyalgia
Motor neuron disease
Multiple sclerosis
Various psychiatric disorders (schizophrenia, endogenous depression, pre senile dementia)
Nutritional deficiencies (B_{12}, folic acid, iron)
Thyroid disorders
Diabetes
Systemic lupus erythematosis (SLE)
Rheumatoid arthritis
Coeliac disease
Crohn's disease
Chronic active hepatitis
Chronic pancreatitis
Coronary artery disease
Pleurisy, other lung conditions (especially if chest symptoms are severe)
Various chronic infections: TB, infectious mononucleosis, Lyme disease, AIDS
Various tropical infections – e.g. amoebic dysentery, bilharzia
Other chronic conditions causing fatigue and ill health, such as cancer.

Investigations

(1) General investigations for all suspected ME patients

Serial weight measurements
Serial a.m. and p.m. temperature measurements
Complete blood count and differential WBC
Serum electrolytes
Blood glucose, creatinine, calcium, phosphate, liver function tests
Plasma viscocity
Creatinine phosphokinase
C reactive protein
Thyroid hormone tests
Autoantibodies profile.

Serology:

EB virus antibodies
Viral capsid antigen (VCA)
EB virus nuclear antigen (EBNA)
ASO and ADBA titres
Antibodies to cytomegalovirus and toxoplasma
ELISA IgM to Coxsackie B virus
Antibodies to hepatitis A and B (depending on history) and for Lyme disease (caused by Borrelia burgdoferi).

(2) More specialized tests

Tensilon test (for myesthenia gravis)
Muscle enzymes
Electrocardiograph (ECG), chest X-ray
T lymphocyte subsets
Muscle biopsy

Electromyogram
Enterovirus protein (EPI).

Results that are Suggestive of ME

Positive C reactive protein, positive IgM to Coxsackie, ratio of T4:T8 lymphocytes reduced.

Bibliography

Acheson, E. D. (1959), 'The clinical syndrome variously called Benign Myalgic Encephalomyelitis, Iceland disease, and Epidemic Neuromyesthenia', *American Journal of Medicine*, vol. 26, pp. 569–95.

Archard, L. C., Behan, P. O., Bell, E. J., Bowles, N. E., Doyle, N. (1988), 'Post viral fatigue syndrome: persistence of enterovirus RNA in muscle and elevated creatine kinase', *Journal of the Royal Society of Medicine*, vol. 81, pp. 326–9.

Arnold, D. L., Bone, P. J., Radda, A. K., Styles, P., Taylor, D. J. (1984), 'Excessive intracellular acidosis of skeletal muscle on exercise in a patient with post-viral exhaustion/fatigue syndrome', *Lancet*, vol. i, pp. 1367–9.

Behan, P. O., Behan, M. H., Bell, E. J. (1985), 'The postviral fatigue syndrome – an analysis of the findings in 50 cases', *Journal of Infection*, vol. 10, pp. 211–22.

Bell, E. J., McCartney, R. A., Riding, M. H. (1988), 'Coxsackie B virus and myalgic encephalomyelitis', *Journal of the Roya Society of Medicine*, vol. 81, pp. 329–31.

Briggs, M., Fox, J., Tedder, R. S. (1988), 'Prevalence of HHV6 in infants and older children', *Lancet*, vol. i, p. 1059.

Buchwald, D., Sullivan, J. L., Komaroff, A. L. (1987), 'Frequenc of "chronic active Epstein-Barr virus infection" in a genera medical practice', *Journal of the American Medical Association* vol. 257, no. 17, pp. 2303–7.

Calder, B. D., Warnock, P. J., McCartney, R. A., Bell, E. J. (1987 'Coxsackie B viruses and the post-viral syndrome: a pros pective study in general practice', *Journal of the Royal College General Practitioners*, vol. 37, pp. 11–14.

Chaitow, L. (1985), *Candida Albicans* (Thorsons).

Crook, W. G. (1986), *The Yeast Connection* (Professional Books).

Davis, A. (1979), *Let's Get Well* (Allen & Unwin).

Davies, S. and Stewart, A. (1987), *Nutritional Medicine* (Pan).

Dowsett, E. G. (1988), 'Human enteroviral infections', *Journal Hospital Infection*, vol. 11, pp. 103–15.

Ganong, W. F. (1983), *Review of Medical Physiology* (Lange).

Gibran, K. (1926), *The Prophet* (Heinemann).

Gray, J. A. (1984), 'Some long-term sequelae of Coxsackie B virus infection', *Journal of the Royal College of General Practitioners*, vol. 84, pp. 3–6.

Hamblin, T. J., Hussain, J., Akbar, A. N., Tang, Y. C., Smith, J. L., Jones, D. B. (1983), 'Immunological reason for chronic ill health after infectious mononucleosis', *British Medical Journal*, vol. 287, pp. 85–7.

Holmes, G. P. *et al.* (1988), 'Chronic fatigue syndrome: a working case definition', *Annals of Internal Medicine*, vol. 108, pp. 387–9.

Ho-Yen, D. (1987), *Better Recovery from Viral Illnesses* (Dodona Books, Old Schoolhouse, Kirkhill, Inverness, IV5 7TE).

Ho-Yen, D., Carrington, D., Armstrong, A. A. (1988), 'Myalgic encephalomyelitis and alpha-interferon', *Lancet*, vol. i, p. 125.

Jamal, G. A. and Hansen, S. (1985), 'Electrophysiological studies in the post-viral fatigue syndrome', *Journal of Neurology, Neurosurgery and Psychiatry*, vol. 48, pp. 691–4.

Jamal, G. A. and Hansen, S. (1988), 'Postviral fatigue syndrome', *British Medical Journal*, vol. 296, pp. 1067–8.

Krueger, G. R. F., Koch, B., Ablashi, D. V. (1987), 'Persistent fatigue and depression in patient with antibody to human B-lymphotropic virus', *Lancet*, vol. ii, p. 36.

Linde, A., Hammarstrom, L., Smith, C. I. E. (1988), 'Ig G subclass deficiency and chronic fatigue syndrome', *Lancet*, vol. i, pp. 885–6.

Lloyd, A., Wakefield, D., Boughton, C., Dwyer, J. (1988), 'What is myalgic encephalomyelitis?', *Lancet*, vol. i, p. 1286.

McEvedy, C. P. and Beard, A. W. (1970), 'Concept of benign myalgic encephalomyelitis', *British Medical Journal*, vol. 1, pp. 11–15.

Mackarness, R. (1976), *Not All in the Mind* (Pan).

Mackarness, R. (1980), *Chemical Victims* (Pan).

Mowbray, J. F. (1988), 'Viruses and neuropsychiatric disorders', *Journal of the Royal Society of Medicine*, vol. 81, pp. 311–12.

Mowbray, J. F., Yousef, G. E., Bell, E. J., Mann, G. F., Smith, D. G., Murugesan, V., McCartney, R. A. (1988), 'Chronic enterovirus infection in patients with postviral fatigue syndrome', *Lancet*, vol. i, pp. 146–9.

Mukherjee, T. M., Smith, K., Maros, K. (1987), 'Abnormal red blood cell morphology in myalgic encephalomyelitis', *Lancet*, vol. ii, pp. 328–9.

Murdoch, J. C. (1987), 'Myalgic encephalomyelitis (ME) syndrome – an analysis of the clinical findings in 200 cases', *New Zealand Family Physician*, Autumn 1987, pp. 51–4.

Ott, J. N. (1976), *Health and Light* (Pocket Books: USA).

Pauling, L. (1986), *How To Live Longer and Feel Better* (W. H. Freeman).

Ramsay, A. M. (1986), *Postviral Fatigue Syndrome* (Gower Medical Publishing).

Randolph, T. G. and Moss, R. W. (1980), *Allergies, your Hidden Enemy* (Thorsons).

Simonton, O. C., Matthews-Simonton, S., Creighton, J. L. (1981), *Getting Well Again* (Bantam Books).

Snell, R. S. (1980), *Clinical Neuroanatomy* (Little, Brown & Co.).

Southern, P. and Oldstone, M. B. A. (1986), 'Medical consequences of persistent viral infection', *New England Journal of Medicine*, vol. 314, no. 6, pp. 359–66.

Wakefield, D. and Lloyd A. (1987), 'Pathophysiology of myalgic encephalitis', *Lancet*, vol. ii, pp. 918–19.

Wakefield, D., Lloyd, A., Dwyer, J. (1988), 'Human herpes virus 6 and myalgic encephalomyelitis', *Lancet*, vol. i, p. 1059.

Williams, R. J. and Kalita, D. K. (1977), *A Physician's Handbook of Orthomolecular Medicine* (Keats).

Wookey, C. (1986), *Myalgic Encephalomyelitis: Post-viral Fatigue Syndrome and How to Cope With It* (Croom Helm).

Yonge, R. P. (1988), 'Magnetic resonance muscle studies: implications for psychiatry', *Journal of the Royal Society of Medicine* vol. 81, pp. 322–5.

Ziff, S. (1984), *The Toxic Time Bomb – Mercury/Amalgam Dental Fillings* (Thorsons).

Index

KEEP MOVING, KEEP YOUNG
Gentle Yoga Exercises for the Elderly £5.95

Here, at last, is an exercise programme designed specifically for those of advancing years, which provides a sound, sensible and enjoyable way of keeping fit and mobile.

This practical, illustrated guide, shows the benefits and enjoyment of gentle yoga-based exercise and relaxation whatever your age or limitations. It is also invaluable for those recuperating from illness and the disabled.

The approach is positive with the accent on what you can achieve. No special equipment or clothing is needed; the basic exercises are performed seated or standing with a chair for support and are listed conveniently working down from head to toes. KEEP MOVING, KEEP YOUNG can be dipped into for specific help – an aching back, arthritic hands – or you can follow the progressive half-hour programmes to work out routines individually or with your group.

Margaret Graham is especially qualified to write this book. She has lived and worked among a lively elderly community for many years and holds the teaching diploma of the British Wheel of Yoga.

THE BOOK OF STRESS SURVIVAL
How to Relax and Live Positively
Alix Kirsta
£7.95 paperback
£12.95 hardback

The Book of Stress Survival is the most useful and comprehensive reference available on stress management. Not only does it examine the causes and effects of stress, it also shows how to pinpoint and reduce the stress in your life. With beautiful illustrations and clear step-by-step instructions, *The Book of Stress Survival* takes you through meditation and relaxation exercises to yoga and massage – essential skills for developing a stress-free lifestyle.

HOMOEOPATHY – THE FAMILY HANDBOOK
An easily understood guide to the selection and use of homoeopathic medicines £3.95

Homoeopathy is practised by doctors all over the world and is generally recognised as an inherently safe form of medication, even for young children.

This Handbook provides a clear and easily understood introduction to the subject, presenting homoeopathy in such a way that it can be used effectively by all the family for first aid and self-care.

The *Symptoms Guide* enables the reader to identify with ease the most suitable remedy for the treatment of common ailments and conditions. The Handbook also provides helpful advice about Homoeopathic practice and lists hospitals, organisations, publications and other sources of useful information.

An essential and valuable book for the newcomer to Homoeopathy.

THE FOOD ALLERGY PLAN
A Working Doctor's Self-Help guide to New Medical Discoveries £4.50
Keith Mumby MB, ChB

The Food Allergy Plan, written by an internationally respected allergy and nutrition expert, takes you step by step through the unmasking of hidden allergies that may spoil your life. Here, at last, may be the answer to many conditions which have failed to respond to drug treatment. A hidden allergy may be responsible for any number of serious illnesses – migraine, colitis, asthma, depression, obesity, dermatitis – as well as a number of minor complaints such as abdominal bloating, mouth ulcers, itchy eyes, palpitations, panic attacks and catarrh.

This remarkable book helps you identify and eliminate those foods from your diet which are causing you physical distress. Doctor Mumby's many successful cases, frequently featured in the media, show how amazing recoveries are achievable by a simple change of diet.

This fully revised, updated edition includes a new chapter on Candida Albicans and is a working doctor's plan for identifying hidden food allergies that may be denying you optimum health. Within weeks, even days, you could be free from chronic or recurring ill-health. Hundreds and thousands of cases from all over the world prove it works.